Depression, Bipolar and Heroin:
Lessons Learned from Losing My Brother to Addiction

Blake LeVine, MSW

Printed by CreateSpace, an Amazon.com company.

Contents

Preface i

1: Breathing.. 1

2: Working Out... 11

3: Family... 17

4: Ways to Deal with Loneliness 25

5: Begin Again 31

6: Fear 37

7: Developing a Positive Attitude.............. 45

8: Embracing Change 53

9: The Longer Road 59

10: Your Inner Fire 67

11: Sharing and Giving 75

12: Choosing Faith over Darkness............. 83

13: Letting Go of the Old You..................... 89

14: Concrete Action 95

15: Listen To Your Heart 103

16: Pass the Test 109

17: A New Outcome...................................... 115

18: Depression and Addiction 121

19: Lemons into Lemonade......................... 127

20: Your New Start.. 131

21: A Final Lesson... 135

Thank You 139

Words of Wisdom from Blake...................... 143

Resources..145

Books by Blake LeVine 147

Films by Blake LeVine..147

Blake's Web Sites..147

Speaking Events 147

About The Author 149

Our Gift to You..151

Preface

I recently lost my 27-year-old brother to heroin addiction. I live with bipolar disorder, and almost lost everything to it.

When you struggle with addiction *and* mental illness, life is a blur. You feel lost, alone, different. Darkness is everywhere. I've written this book to guide you along a path that leads to light, hope, and healing.

While living in New York in 2001, I watched the Twin Towers fall. It was a smoky, dark and scary time. In the days and weeks that followed, I witnessed the healing that took place. We came together to rebuild our city and move forward.

Dealing with addiction and mental illness should be handled in the same way. You need to take down the broken foundation, build a strong new base and, slowly, rise again. You have to begin making better choices.

Before my brother died I was called to help those who suffer from mental illness and addiction. While working with these patients, I noticed that rehab facilities often fail to end addiction. I wondered why. Most people in rehab don't want to die. They don't work so hard to rebuild their lives, while believing that they're wasting their time. It would be much easier for them to get stoned every day than to make the effort to turn their lives around.

So why doesn't rehab always work? And why do some of us put our lives at risk by playing Russian roulette with drugs and alcohol in the first place? Is it because of a genetic disorder, stress, pain – or is it something else? As I continued to work with these patients, I began to find some of the answers.

Pain lurks behind all drug abuse. Pain caused by feeling lost or "different." Pain from always feeling confused or angry. Pain that is not easily or quickly overcome. Pain that requires a long-term, committed, focused, disciplined and thought-out process of living differently to relieve it.

This book will change you – if you let it. I've written it to help you find healing and the courage to believe in yourself, and in God. It will enable you to learn all of the life lessons God has shared with me about addiction and mental illness. Addicts, the mentally ill, families who live with these problems (including parents, spouses and children), teachers, medical professionals – anyone who wants to learn more about these issues – will benefit from reading it.

In recent years, all of us have watched a heroin epidemic take the lives of some of the brightest lights in our society. I pray that the words on these pages will give you a better understanding of the problems – and their solutions. If only one life is transformed by it, this book will be a success. May God bless you as you begin your spiritual transformation.

Those who suffer from bipolar disorder swing between states of extreme excitement and complete hopelessness. We all need pure joy and happiness, but when we push ourselves too far in either direction, problems develop. I've seen capable, creative, energetic and loving clients who suffer from bipolar disorder, work towards a goal, only to burn out before they reach it. I've also seen others, who once felt passion and bliss, trapped in a despair that robs them of every bit of energy.

Living with mental illness in a healthy way can be a complex and (sometimes) dramatic undertaking. Living with addiction can consume all of your energy, just surviving and staying sober.

Together, mental illness and addiction put a huge obstacle in the way of those who suffer from them. This book teaches you how to systematically trace the origins of the problem, so that you can break it down and move forward.

Each of the 21 chapters describes how to overcome mental illness and addiction in holistic ways. As a life coach for those who suffer from addiction and mental illness, my job is to create a roadmap to help them rebuild and move forward. I've seen clients make adjustments and slowly learn to be peaceful, balanced and drug-free.

My brother's death enabled me to experience the pain and loss that families suffer when a loved one dies from addiction. If your life is saved by what you learn from this book, he didn't die in vain. Beneath his addiction was a beautiful soul – warm and compassionate – who loved life. He snowboarded, danced, traveled, attended nudist resorts, surfed and rode dirt bikes. He wasn't afraid to try anything that he thought might be a "rush." I'm more reserved than he was, but I'm happy that he had so many adventures and was always willing to try new things. He taught me to be open, and to accept who I am.

Take another look at the photo on the front cover of this book. That's my brother Adam. It was taken in the mountains above Beverly Hills the last time I saw him alive. He came to visit me in Los Angeles, and was considering moving there. I hoped to take him under my wing – to be a positive influence on him – but he decided not to stay. Instead, he moved to Vermont, taking a job at a ski resort.

I spoke with him on the phone for over an hour on the day he died. He told me that, for the first time in his life, he felt that he fit in with the people around him – his friends and co-workers. I was the last person in our family to speak with him.

I'll always love my brother – my only brother – and feel blessed to have been in his life. I hope this book reaches other addicts and their families, and helps them to learn how to defeat their demons.

Note: All of the case examples in this book have been altered to protect the privacy of Blake's clients. Names and other details have been altered or omitted. These examples are included as teaching tools, and are true to the treatment concepts examined in this book.

1: Breathing

It's easy to tell someone to breathe, but it's not always easy for them to do it. We're often so swept up in our emotions that we become anxious. We might be nervous about our finances, careers, addiction, or things that we have lost. We feel like we can't breathe.

James

James was a young man from a rich family from Denver. He lived in Los Angeles and struggled to stay sober. He was addicted to crack cocaine. He said it helped him to escape the moment and forget his past.

As a child, James was abused by his aunt. The experience made him feel dirty. He told his family, but they didn't believe him. He grew up feeling awkward, and had relationship difficulties. He frequently had sex with women, but didn't enjoy it. He'd begin relationships but would become hostile (and sometimes violent) towards the women. Most of the relationships ended with him no longer speaking to them.

During our work together, James realized that his aggression towards women resulted from the anger he felt towards his aunt. He applied his feelings about her abuse to every new relationship with a woman. We worked hard to help him understand that his past could continue to define him forever, or he could change.

I told James to take ten deep breaths whenever he started to feel upset or angry. I also told him to buy a punching bag and install it in his garage. Whenever he began to feel upset he would take ten deep breaths, then go to the garage and hit the bag 100 times (or hit it until he had no energy left). He told me that when he did this, all of his rage drained away. Before he began treatment, he'd become angry and violent, or would sneak away to smoke crack, whenever he was upset. By breathing and hitting the bag he was able to reduce his frustration and stop hurting women.

Quinn

Meditation is a good way for us to center ourselves and to quiet inner turmoil. A young woman named Quinn came in for a session to work on her bipolar disorder. She reported that she often felt lonely, and too unhealthy to be in a relationship. Quinn was beautiful, with short brown hair, big blue eyes and a soft smile. Her family was poor, and her dad left when she was six. She'd always been afraid of being in a relationship, and suffered from stomach disorders. She visited the doctor frequently.

Together, we reviewed her personal history. Quinn admitted that being abandoned by her dad caused her to distrust men. During her frequent childhood sicknesses, her mom and grandma gave her extra attention. She learned that love was not easy to find, and that manipulating her mom in this way resulted in them spending more time together.

Quinn built a negative cycle: she got sick, received attention, missed school and then would not want to return to school. She had trouble connecting with other children, especially girls. She liked boys, and secretly wanted a boyfriend. But when a boy would get close to her, she would get sick or run away. This left her isolated, depressed and alone. To cope, she began smoking marijuana every day. She was diagnosed with bipolar disorder and addictions. Day-to-day living had become a major problem for her.

Quinn had trouble holding a job but, as we continued to work together, we discovered that she was a gifted teacher. She was very patient with children and loved to work with them. She had previously taught part-time at a preschool – her favorite subject was reading. Together, we discovered that she had the desire, and the ability, to be a reading teacher and tutor.

Quinn started using a breathing and meditation technique that I call *Finding Peace for the Day*. Rising at 7am, she would sit quietly on a yoga mat with no interruptions for an hour. No television, phone, or anything else that would distract her. She would perform a series of exercises that included five minutes of breathing normally with her eyes closed. During this time Quinn would tell herself to let go and not think of anything. During those five minutes her thoughts and fears diminished.

Her next step was to repeat affirmations for ten minutes. In this part of the technique, the patient focuses on three items he or she wants to believe. Quinn's items were "I am calm. I am a good teacher. I am healthy, physically and mentally." The three items are repeated over and over again for ten minutes. The repetition helps you to believe that the items are true – that they describe your reality. After several days of repeating affirmations for ten minutes, your psyche begins to accept them.

The third step in the technique is to chant for ten minutes. My grandmother (who was a psychic) shared this with me. You calmly spread your arms out and say "Om, Om, Om, Om." Do this for ten minutes, letting the energy flow through your lungs and body, while releasing all fears or past pain.

The fourth step is what I call a 30-minute "awake sleep." Sit calmly on your mat and do not allow yourself to be distracted. Keep your eyes closed for 30 minutes. Try to prevent any fears from entering your mind. Think of the word "love." In your head, say "Love, Love, Love." Wait to see what God (or "the source") brings to you. It might be words, a thought, the answer to a problem or some other form of knowledge.

When you begin this technique, time will pass slowly. You might be uncomfortable, and will want it to stop. Eventually, you'll grow to love this calm and peaceful time. If you have children or are married it might be difficult to be alone for an hour. I suggest using earplugs or headphones to tune out any commotion in your home.

By practicing this technique every day, Quinn experienced a shift in her energy. She gained the courage to take two important life steps. One was to earn a degree in teaching by completing a program she had previously dropped out of. She also posted a profile on a dating website called *Plenty of Fish*. She started going on dates and began to accept that not all men are bad. She forgave her father for leaving her family and learned to let go of the anger and pain she felt towards him. After several years, she was married and had a successful career as a teacher. The genuine love of her husband and her job success enabled her to let go of her marijuana addiction. Quinn is now a vibrant, positive and beautiful human being.

One of the main reasons for using these techniques is to center your brain. When I was younger, I would wake up with fearful thoughts. I'd think about my problems, and worried about how things would turn out for me. As a result, I'd lose my ability to live in the moment. I've learned that taking time to focus on breathing early in the day has a number of benefits, including beginning your day on a healthy and positive note.

Here's another tip which has provided me with a wonderful amount of increased energy. When I was in college, I would wake up and think that I needed five more minutes of sleep. I would even set my alarm clock to wake me one hour before I had to get up, so that I go back to sleep for five more minutes, five more minutes, etc. I dreaded the time when I finally had to stay awake for the rest of the day! It began to weigh on me. I was starting my days in a negative state of mind.

During this time, I started listening to Houston pastor Joel Osteen. One of his sermons focused on the importance of beginning each day in an encouraged and happy way. So I tried an experiment: the moment I woke up I said "Thank you God for allowing me to wake up. Thank you God for allowing me to be healthy enough to get up and do my work. Thank you for making today a great day." I began feeling happy the moment I said this. In my heart, I really was grateful to be alive and able to breathe, walk, talk and listen. I realized that my brother wasn't able to do these things, and that they were blessings that I shouldn't take for granted.

Another key step was to get up when the alarm went off. Immediately. Those five extra minutes were toxic because they allowed me to resist embracing the new day. Expressing simple gratitude and praying while I'm waking up makes me feel more alive and motivated, looking forward to whatever comes next.

I was a cigarette smoker during my teenage years. I thought it helped me to make friends, remove stress and stay calm. After a few years of smoking I noticed that my breathing and health were changing, and not for the better. I began to get nosebleeds and found it difficult to exercise. I was in my early 20s, but I became winded and tired easily.

At the same time I observed my mother-in-law's struggles. Her name is Randy. She was dealing with a lot of stress. She and her husband would often argue, which made her anxious. She would pick at her skin and smoke constantly – I believe it was her escape. During the first few years that I dated my wife, I saw Randy get sicker. When it became hard for her to breathe, she began to depend on an oxygen tank. The simplest physical tasks became difficult for her. During a family trip to Las Vegas, we wanted to go to dinner, which required a short walk to the restaurant. Randy couldn't walk more than a few feet without getting tired and winded. She had to make several stops and it took away her happiness at being with her daughter's family.

As the years passed her health deteriorated. She made frequent trips to the hospital to for breathing support. During one of her hospital stays her doctor called and told us to come right away. My wife remained with Randy during her last few days of life, soothing and caring for her. She later described the experience as "watching someone drown."

I'm sad that my mother-in-law will never meet her grandson. She was the only family member in the room when my daughter was born. We experienced many wonderful times together. The pain my wife feels over her loss continues to this day. I've shared this story with you as a way of talking about addiction and smoking, and the pain and loss they inflict on families.

When I worked at a rehab facility, I noticed that most patients were heavy smokers. During the five daily smoke breaks, nearly all of the 40 clients would chain-smoke. I knew that this would eventually kill them. Even if they overcame their addictions to opiates, alcohol or cocaine, they wouldn't be free of their cigarette addiction. Their cravings were so strong that many would chew tobacco secretly.

I know how hard it is to overcome drug and alcohol addiction. Smoking can be just as hard to quit. I quit and relapsed three times before I was finally able to stop for good. I know that I can never smoke even one cigarette ever again. It's been more than ten years since I stopped. My breathing is stronger, I have more energy and I'm healthier in general.

The hardest part of quitting was the beginning. During my first four days without cigarettes I was a jerk. Angry, nasty, rude. A terror to be near. I saw that it would be best if I was alone during the early days of my withdrawal. After I got through them, it became easier.

I understood that I could never have another cigarette – not one. You are either all in or all out with the smoking addiction. I knew that if I smoked I would eventually hurt my wife, just like her mother did. I promised myself that I would not let that happen and would stay healthy.

Are you ready to learn to breathe? Are you willing to stop putting toxins in your body and to start feeling your emotions? Many people allow their frustrations to get deep into their hearts and take away their joy. Don't be one of them.

Timmy

Journaling is a healthy way to release whatever's on your mind. Buy a simple notebook or a beautiful journal – it doesn't matter. In it, write down what you want to work on and record your feelings. Be candid with yourself. Write exactly what you think and feel.

I worked with a man named Timmy. He was 40 and divorced. His wife left him due to his alcohol addiction. He said he felt anger about his parents and childhood. Timmy struggled to share exactly what bothered him. I asked him to get a journal and write about what he felt, including the anger. The next week he returned with over 20 pages of thoughts, drawings and writing.

Timmy's journal told how he felt his parents had created darkness in his life. They abused alcohol, and were often hostile towards him. His dad hit him and treated him as if he was worthless. Timmy also wrote about his brother leaving home at 16 and never speaking to any of the family again.

Timmy had been frustrated since he was a boy. He never let go of these emotions. He became very angry, and thought that drinking calmed him down. He wrote that he repeated the pattern and abused his wife. He understood why she left him, and realized that he wasn't healthy enough to be a good husband.

We worked together to help him learn to breathe and let go of his past. He needed to remove his anger and pain in order to stop drinking. Timmy attended an outpatient rehab program, went to Alcoholics Anonymous meetings and worked with me.

When he stopped drinking, everything came down on him like an avalanche. He had money problems, job struggles, and he felt horrible. I encouraged him to slow down, breathe deeply, and take things one moment at a time. He got through the first week and began to truly live. For the first time in years, he began to feel. His emotions were heavy and hard. Timmy was no longer hiding and had nothing to numb his thoughts.

Timmy expressed what he felt through journaling. He took his blue, three-ring notebook with him wherever he went. Whenever he felt nervous or upset, he wrote about it. Timmy said the notebook became his new outlet. Instead of reaching for a drink, he wrote. He re-read what he had written in his journal at the end of each week. When he did, he saw how he was transforming and owning his thoughts.

Timmy remains in recovery. He found friends in AA who understood his past and his addiction. Eventually he found a good job at a construction company and started to date a beautiful woman who is also in recovery. He says that he still takes time to write in his journal each day, and to breathe.

Blake LeVine

2: Working Out

Our bodies need to move. To work. As a child I played baseball, tennis, street hockey and basketball. I always loved a good workout. But as I grew older, my patterns changed. I focused on my responsibilities, and family concerns became my priority. My career and the care of my two children became more important than exercise. I ate comfort foods to numb my feelings.

Two years ago I was overweight, had high blood pressure and stomach problems. I was only 33, but knew that I couldn't continue to live as I had. I made a small start by making a big decision: I would walk for 30 minutes to an hour each day at 4pm. I promised myself that no matter what was happening, I would do it. My wife loves going to the gym, but I don't like it. I feel self-conscious and don't like being so close to others who are working out. I decided to walk around my neighborhood instead.

We lived in the "Miracle Mile" section of Los Angeles. During my walk I saw the Hollywood sign and the mountains. I also glanced at the beautiful plants and trees my neighbors had planted in their yards. I made the effort to smile at everyone I passed. This hour in the sun was good for me and filled me with natural vitamins.

My first month of walking was the most difficult, because I was lazy. I made excuses, including being tired, having work to do or just not wanting to go. I pushed through them and continued to go each day. I lost weight and felt lighter. My digestion improved and I ate healthier. I had more energy and felt better overall.

Over time, I lost 30 pounds. These days, I work out every day and I love it. The fresh air and the release of energy are healing. I recently started running, since I felt extra energy and my body is stronger than it was when I started walking. I walk and run further than I've ever been able to in my life. I watch my food intake and make better dietary choices. In the past, I ate fast food, lots of bread and heavy meals. Now I eat less – only enough to feel satisfied. Here's a healthy tip: only buy what's good for you to eat. If I have food in the house that is unhealthy I'm likely to eat it in a weak moment.

Jamie

I started working with Jamie, who was 30 and had a long history of neglecting her body. In her early years she was overweight and was ridiculed for it. She ate to relieve the pain she felt when other children teased her. In her teens she began vomiting to stop gaining weight. This caused her to have a number of health problems. As she grew up, she continued to battle weight issues. She defined herself by what the scale said.

Jamie and I were open with each other about how this was harming her. I told her that if she didn't care for her body it would break down. In addition to being overweight, she was addicted to Adderall. She began to take it for ADD, but eventually used it to lose weight. Her problems persisted, and her doctor said that her heart was showing the effects of a rapid heartbeat and hypertension.

As I worked with Jamie, she said that she was afraid to change. For as long as she remembered, her weight was the focal point of her life: she cared more about it than anything else. She admitted that if she didn't correct her patterns, the odds were that her life would be a short one.

I knew that Jamie needed to work on both the mental and physical aspects of her life. When we spoke about sports and exercise, she said she felt very little energy and hated working out. She mentioned that she played tennis as a child and was pretty good at it, so I encouraged her to buy a racket and take a lesson. Jamie signed up with a local tennis pro and went to the public courts. She started with 30 minutes of hitting and began to feel happy as she worked out.

Jamie indicated that when she played tennis, she forgot about her problems – her weight and the stress that came with it. She began to feel more alive and connected to the world. As the weeks passed she started playing four times a week. She joined a non-competitive doubles game with three other women. They became friends, relaxing and discussing their lives after their matches.

Jamie let go of her weight fixation. She started eating better, as it helped her play tennis at a higher level. She also worked with her psychiatrist to stop abusing Adderall. Jamie realized that many of her problems were in her head. When she combined therapy, exercise, friendship and healthy eating, her life improved in big ways.

It's been several years since Jamie began to rewrite her story. Today she is healthier, more connected with nature and less nervous. She let go of her biggest problem and allowed herself to heal. She enjoys working, playing tennis, hiking and being with friends. She eats to live; she doesn't live to eat. It's clear to her that food is an energy source and weight is only a number. She knows that everyone has a different body type and that genetics play a big part in appearance. Jamie became her own best friend and, for the first time, accepted herself.

I'm often asked why working out makes such a big impact. It's because each part of our mind and body was created to be useful. When you sit around all day, the body holds onto too much energy. Without proper outlets, the energy turns toxic and becomes harmful. When you feel pain, often it is because you haven't released energy properly. Many of us work in offices five days a week, for 40 hours, sitting in a chair. We aren't meant to be glued to a seat for that long.

As a writer and therapist, I often sit for long periods of time. If I neglect myself and sit too long, I begin to feel pain. To prevent this from happening, or to relieve whatever pain I may be feeling, I stand up, stretch, bounce and sometimes take a short walk after therapy sessions. This allows me to release my energy and not stagnate.

Farah

Farah, one of my clients, worked long hours sitting at a desk. She would come home in pain and drink wine to relax and relieve her sore back. When I told her about my stretching routine, she laughed. She asked how she could she do that on the job (she worked for a high-powered law firm). If her bosses saw her bouncing around and stretching they would think that she was crazy.

We laughed. She had a point. It might seem strange to start bouncing around a business office. Imagine a police officer in uniform bouncing around his desk. Or the workers at the DMV. I agreed that she needed to behave properly at work.

I asked Farrah where she went when she needed privacy. She said she was allowed time for breaks and was able to go outside. I asked if there was a park near her office. Farrah told me about a beautiful park with palm trees, flowers, benches and a children's playground. We decided she should go there once a day during her lunch break. For 20 minutes she would stretch, practice breathing, and just stand up. She would use the time to break away from all of that sitting.

Farah also agreed to stretch for 15 minutes when she came home from work, and to jog for 45 minutes. This additional hour would help her to process all that had happened during the day. When she began to do it, she stopped drinking. Her previous pattern of coming home and having a drink was replaced by exercise. When she finished jogging she would shower, eat dinner and relax. This enabled her to end her addiction and eliminate her back pain.

You need to move. I challenge you to start doing so today. Stretch, take a short walk, go to the gym, practice yoga, play tennis or basketball, run – do something that makes your body work. Change is hard and good results don't come easily. I've found that not thinking, just taking action, is often the remedy for laziness. Don't just think about working out. What are you going to do today to be healthy? Whatever your answer is, find the time and make it happen. If you start, and stay with it, you'll see your health improve.

Blake LeVine

3: Family

The loss of my brother to heroin addiction impacted my entire family. A landslide of change swept into our lives. But it also helped us understand how important life is and that we need to enjoy the time we share while we have it. I want to tell you about my family and how they've helped me rebuild my life.

My dad was 32 and my mother was 16 when they met. They moved to New York City and lived a fast-paced life of drugs and partying. There is a famous story about my 9-months-pregnant mother dancing the night away at Studio 54 and having me early the next day.

When I was a child, my parents began to fight and ended up filing for divorce. Their legal battle was brutal. As part of the final decree, my dad was allowed only limited supervised visitation, which made him furious. My mother claimed that he abused me. He vehemently denied it. I was so young at the time that I don't remember much about it now.

One day as I walked with my mom and her friend on the upper east side of Manhattan, a car pulled up. My mom and her friend were knocked to the ground and I was kidnapped by my dad.

He took me to South Carolina. I was lost and confused. Again and again I asked him where my mom was. He allowed me to call her once a month. Whenever I called, I could hear her crying as we spoke. Mom begged me to tell her where I was, but all I could say was that I was in the brown house down the street. I was too young to understand that I was hours away from her.

My dad and I bonded during the 10 months we were together in South Carolina. We fished, ate French fries at Wendy's, and had fun at a local playground.

My mother was devastated but knew that she couldn't give in to depression and sadness if we were to be reunited. Just when she was ready to give up, she found me. A private detective she had hired located me at a nursery school, even though my hair had been dyed white-blond. When we were reunited, my mom didn't recognize me until I screamed "Mommy I love you." We went to court the next day.

My dad was arrested, but since it had been a *parental* kidnapping it was viewed less harshly by the court (this was during the early 1980s). In her heart, my mother knew that my dad loved me more than anything. She realized that if she took me away from him completely, she'd always be afraid that he would kidnap me again – and that he might kill her. So she allowed him to be in my life.

I lived with my mother during the week and stayed with my dad on the weekends. Mom and I moved into a tiny apartment on Staten Island, and she began working as a school bus driver at my preschool. She met my stepfather, Marc, and they fell in love. He was a warm, kind man who was wonderful with children. He accepted me and became a second father to me. They later married and had two children.

I developed strong connections to my step-siblings. My stepbrother Adam was a beautiful soul who built amazing things out of wood – beginning when he was a child. He built skateboard ramps, created art, and was always on the lookout for adventure. I loved him so much, and felt like I had a best friend for life. We played sports, traveled together and had a lot of fun.

As a college graduation gift, I took Adam to Hollywood. We stayed at a funky hotel called The Standard on the Sunset Strip.

We went to restaurants, went dancing and had a blast. Adam was in his addiction, so he spent much of the trip at a medical marijuana dispensary. His also went to the Hustler shop and bought a lot of funny/sexual t-shirts. That's who he was and he wouldn't change for anyone.

My stepsister Chayse, my youngest sibling, is smart, sensitive and stunningly beautiful. I never know what she'll say to me, but she's always honest. Once, as we at lunch, she laughed and told me that I "chew my carrots like a horse." Chayse is a fine athlete – an expert horsewoman – who loves animals and children. We used to fight, but have become best friends.

Chayse has been working on herself in therapy. I introduced her to a friend who broke up with his fiancé. He and Chayse have been dating, and are helping each other to enjoy life.

I have another sister, Natasha, through my dad who also remarried. His new wife, Anna, often fought with him but she's been a great mother to Natasha. Natasha is warm, sweet, shy and beautiful. She's been in a relationship for many years with her high school sweetheart, Reed, who lost both of his parents before he finished college. He and Natasha were together throughout that time.

My birth dad (who kidnapped me) is a genius. He looks like Mick Jagger – many people have asked him if he is with the Rolling Stones. My dad has had many problems but he genuinely loves his children. When I visited him on weekends, we would do whatever I wanted to do. My first dream was to play baseball, so we would play for seven or eight hours a day. When I later decided that I wanted to meet celebrities and get their autographs, he was happy to help me. We spent years finding and meeting famous people. How many dads would wait outdoors in the dead of winter for five hours while their son waited to meet Tom Cruise?

When I was 14, President Clinton invited me to The White House. I had previously met Mother Teresa, Madonna, Michael Jackson, Britney Spears, Frank Sinatra, Margaret Thatcher, seven U.S. presidents, Paul McCartney, Steven Spielberg, Bob Dylan, The Dalai Lama, Bill Cosby, Michael Jordan, and over 4,000 others. My dad and I wrote *OK Dad, You Can Take the Picture: A Young Man's Quest of Autographs of the Famous*, which was published when I was 15.

Something else happened when I was 15: I began to suffer from bipolar hallucinations, delusions and paranoia. I spent time in psychiatric hospitals and lost my friends, family and freedom. When my family visited, they gave me hope – and brought me the special foods that I liked. They never gave up on me. Even though I was getting worse, they didn't stop trying. They spent thousands of dollars on therapists, psychiatrists and anyone who they thought might help me.

My stepdad Marc showered me with kindness and love, even when I was abusive to him. He treated me as his own son, and never gave up hope that I would recover. He had a busy career and two other children, but he stood by my mom's side and kept her hope alive.

My two grandmothers have played a big part in my life. My mom's mother has had enough adventures to fill ten lives. She's been a hippy, psychic, a rock singer, comedienne, writer, belly dancer, snake charmer, mistress to William DeKooning, and the list goes on. She taught me to believe in myself and to take chances. A courageous single Jewish woman, she was not afraid pick up and start over in a new place. She has lived in India, Spain, England and many other countries.

My stepdad's mother, Arlene, is a wonderful human being. She accepted me as her grandchild and has always been there for our family. When we needed money, she helped us out. When I needed a friend, she was there for me. Arlene had a near-fatal stroke at the same time that my brother died. I believe in my heart that she survived because we needed her.

For over a month, we didn't tell Arlene that Adam had died. We wanted her to focus on her recovery, and were worried that telling her might cause another stroke. One day she went to lunch with my mom and wife and asked about Adam. My mom responded by asking her what she thought had happened to him. My grandma said "I think he is dead." Mom asked her if she really wanted to know, and she said yes. So they told her, confirming her worst fears.

My family is large one, and is what I call "healthily dysfunctional." We all have our problems, including me. But together we celebrate the good times and help each other through the dark ones. I wouldn't have survived my mental illness without the love of my family. Their love shows me why I'm in this world.

Recovery from addiction and mental illness often begins with your family. You must learn your family history. For some, this means finding out about family addictions, health problems and other difficulties. I remember a very powerful talk on this topic which continues to resonate with me. The speaker told us that some families have a history of alcoholism going back through many generations. But what would happen if someone in that family overcame his or her addiction? That person would change family history! Those who came after that person would be able to say "if he/she stopped drinking, maybe I can too."

All of us can make choices that are different from those made by past generations. When you choose to live a healthy life, you prove what someone from your family can do. My good choices help my children. My wife and I both grew up in homes with a lot of fighting and tension, but our home is peaceful and calm. My two children feel safe and supported. This will help them, as they develop, to be optimistic and confident. We've replaced the old family pattern with a new and better one.

Kelly

Kelly felt that her parents tried to control her and projected their problems onto her. Her mom had social phobia and liked to be alone. Her dad was an alcoholic who feared that Kelly would fall into his addiction. Both parents created an environment of fear and conflict.

Kelly told me that she began to escape at a young age. She tried to be funny, to lighten up the tense situation at home. That didn't work so well. When she got a little older she began to drink heavily and use cocaine. These drugs helped Kelly to relax and forgot about her parents.

Her parents got angry when they found out what she'd been doing and sent her to rehab. She stopped using for a few weeks, but when she came home the environment was still tense and toxic. It wasn't long before Kelly started using again. She felt horrible because she knew it was going to end badly. She was sure that either her parents would kick her out or she'd die.

Instead, she committed to making a transformation. Kelly attended Narcotics Anonymous meetings and found a sponsor. She opened up about her past, and talked about feeling misunderstood. Even though she was funny and popular, that was not how she felt. She saw herself as odd and not good enough.

Kelly never let go of her parents' failures. She knew that her dad had tried to be a comedian, but failed. She thought that if she could be successful, he would be proud of her. It was as if she carried a burden to achieve something that was in his heart, not hers.

We challenged her understanding of the family dynamics at work in her life. Kelly realized that she didn't want a career in the public spotlight. Her true self wanted peace and a simple life. Her dream was to be married with children. She wanted to take care of them and give them the supportive home she never had. I explained to her that she could have this, but only if she overcame her addiction.

For many months, Kelly worked to change her outlook on life, drugs and her family. She began to uncover her true personality – the hidden gem inside her. After a year of recovery, she started dating. A friend from NA had a cousin who also came from a troubled home. He had been in therapy, and was ready to find love. Eventually, they married and built a beautiful, loving home that included three children. Because Kelly worked on herself first, she was ready to find real love, and prepared to build a new life. I'm blessed to have helped her through her troubles so that she could reach the light at the end of the tunnel. I know that you, like Kelly, can rework your life.

None of us pick our parents. It's up to us to accept them, and to learn how to make progress from wherever we begin. Every situation is different, but all of them contain issues that benefit from being addressed. Are you addicted because of your family history? If so, you must work to understand it, then put it behind you. Remember: the people who love you wish that they could get through to you and apologize for the mistakes they've made.

Many of us have children early in our lives, or during a time when we are not doing well. Most parents try their best, but are not always equipped to handle their responsibilities. Create as much support around yourself as you can. It can include NA, AA, a therapist, a sober coach, psychiatrist, sober friends and family who care. "It takes a village" to overcome addiction. When you add allies to your army of healing you have the best chance to win the war on addiction.

4: Ways to Deal with Loneliness

Have you ever been in a room that was filled with people, but you felt alone? Many of my patients have spoken to me about their long-term loneliness. They struggle to make connections, they're easily hurt, and they have trouble with the ups and downs of personal interaction. I've come across these problems time and time again.

In the past, my wife and I sometimes lived in old/small homes in big cities. And sometimes she complained about our living conditions. When she did, I offered encouragement and hope, and tried to cheer her up and/or "fix" the situation.

We eventually settled in Florida and now have a beautiful home. The rooms are large and modern, with stainless steel appliances, marble countertops, a flower-filled backyard and nice neighbors. I expected my wife to say "Wow, I love this home. It's everything that I want." Instead, she told me that she liked the house but hated Florida.

I can't really "fix" our living situation because my wife's unhappiness was never really about the size or features of the house. I had a helpful conversation about this with a friend and his wife. He said they lived in a small apartment when they first started dating. She hated it, and complained to him about it. They eventually got a big house, but she still complains that it doesn't have certain features.

When my wife is unhappy, I feel alone. My main purpose in life is to take care of her and our two children. I used to try to make everything perfect for her and hoped that, by doing so, our life would be great. Now I know that I can't do it and that, sometimes, her negativity is not based on facts.

In our case, our home was not the problem. Not really. Instead, it's a hodgepodge of my wife missing her mom (who died in Florida), her negativity (which has always been there), the anger she feels about not doing well-enough financially, and an overall feeling of not being good enough. She's working on these problems, and I am trying to figure out how to take care of myself while she does. I'm her husband, but it's not my job to "fix" her. I know that she'll have good days, bad days, and some that are in-between.

When a loved one has bipolar disorder or addictions, his or her relationship with you may suffer. When they feel rejected, they may want to get "high" and escape their discomfort. Many addicts are ultra-sensitive (as I am). We're devastated when lovers, friends or family members hurt our feelings. Many of us try to detach or say "the hell with them anyway," and give up on the relationship. I used to end friendships if someone said or did something that hurt me emotionally.

I've learned in my own therapy that even the best of us have bad days and say hurtful things. And so I look at the big picture. With respect to my wife, I remind myself that she's kind, loving, faithful, hard-working, smart, a great mother, good at details. Best of all, she believes in me.

When she's upset, I stop and think before getting angry at her. I look at the situation and do my best to understand it. Her negativity could be due to something like Mothers' Day reminding her of her mom, who passed away three years ago. Whatever it is, or might be, I use it to put her behavior in perspective. Instead of focusing on what she says, I look deeper – at what is not said.

Depression, Bipolar and Heroin

I've learned how to overcome loneliness by changing the situation. Mother's Day was a long day in our family. We spent it with my mom, wife, stepdad, sister, our children and about 15 other relatives at my mother's house. After a long visit, we started on our way home.

My wife was tired and sad about her mom not being with us (even though she didn't say that this was on her mind, I knew that it was). Our seven-month-old son screamed for over an hour in the car. Then my six-year-old daughter began to scream – it was a mess. As we arrived at our house, my wife threatened to leave us. I asked where she would go. She said "I don't know, but somewhere far away from here." Instead of fighting with her (and making her feel worse) I told her that I'd take both kids to Walmart to do our weekly grocery shopping.

I put both kids back in the car and off we went. When we got there, I carried my six-year-old on my shoulders and wheeled the baby in his stroller. I got a huge cart for our food. As we walked through Walmart, the people we passed smiled and laughed. I remained calm as I pushed my screaming baby in the stroller with my left hand and pulled the cart with my right. We went through all 20 aisles and got all of the groceries we needed. As we stood in the checkout line, I prayed that my wife would still be there when we got home.

The checkout line would have moved faster if a blind turtle had been working at the register. I never saw a cashier work so slowly. I decided to buy a bottle of water and have a piece of candy. I gave my daughter a lip balm as she waited patiently. As I started to put my groceries on the counter, another register opened up. I wanted to be patient, but waiting for over an hour with a newborn and a six-year-old is not easy.

I grabbed my groceries and moved to the other register. The cashier was amazed at how relaxed we were. She checked us out, we paid and went home. I didn't know what I'd find when we got there. I listened to religious music in the car and prayed that my wife would be calm.

When we arrived my wife was relaxed and happy to see us! You would never have guessed that an hour earlier she was thinking of running away. Our babysitter was there, ready to help. Together we put the groceries away. Later, my wife got a good night's sleep and woke up the next day in a much better mood. Our life was back to normal.

Days like this can leave me feeling lonely and depressed. But I know that if I had taken a drink or gotten high our problems wouldn't have gone away. Things would have kept on getting worse and we would have had a full-blown drama to deal with.

I once worked with a group of addicts in a 60-day rehab center. During a discussion about loneliness, I asked each of them to share a story about a time when they'd felt alone. Some of them talked about times when a girlfriend cheated on them, a parent fought with them, times when they felt that they had no friends, or the death of someone they loved. They also spoke about how, during these painful times, they would smoke coke, drink alcohol, smoke marijuana blunts, hire a prostitute, or shoot heroin. When they felt lost and alone, getting high enabled them to escape and leave those feelings behind. We talked about how men (the group was made up of adult males), are sensitive too and don't like feeling alone. When we're hurting, we feel as if it's us against the world.

We spoke of ways to deal with loneliness without hurting ourselves. The discussion was a lively one, and some good alternatives were shared. These included finding others who accept you as you are now. These "others" can include people in recovery and family members, including your kids. Even starting a new hobby can help. Once you begin to open yourself up, you'll find others who want to be in your life.

Donny

Donny told me that he was always alone. He worried that the stealing he did to support his heroin addiction made him unlikeable. I told him what I'd learned about this from the late poet, Maya Angelou. She said that there was a time in her life when someone told her that God loved her. She had to hear it a few times before it sank in. When she realized that God loved her just as she is, it was a defining moment. She began to accept herself.

I told Donny that God loves him as he is – including his past and all of his negative behavior. God loves him despite the pain he inflicted on those from whom he stole, and on his family. When I asked Donny if he accepted himself, he said that he was ashamed of himself. It was easier for him to be alone, so he wouldn't have to worry about being picked on or rejected. He told me that being alone was hard, and he was scared to live a life without drugs. He didn't know who he was, and was defined by being a heroin addict. Donny spoke about the core of his heart, which had been hardened by the pain of his life.

I encouraged Donny to look at what was good about him. Other clients said that Donny was patient, giving, a good listener, was not using drugs and tried to help others. I asked Donny how it would feel to believe that God loved him. He thought about it, then said it would mean he'd have to love himself. I told him that if he didn't love himself he couldn't love anyone else. Donny thought about this and began to change.

On the day that he left rehab Donny and I had a heart-to-heart talk. He understood that his life was changing. He had stayed off drugs for 60 days and made a new start. I asked him about our discussion about God and his self-worth. Donny said that he'd thought about it, and began to take inventory of his life. He felt, for the first time, that he deserved to have friends. He made two close friends in rehab and exchanged phone numbers with them. He said that he would attend NA with them.

Donny connected with others and accepted God. He said that it energized him to know God loves him. His courage enabled him to break the cycle of isolation and loneliness.

There are times when I want to be alone, but I know that I have gifts that other people need. When you're with others, you have an opportunity to create love, peace, inspiration – and community. We all need others: stay close to them and allow them to get close to you.

5: Begin Again

One of the most complicated aspects of addiction and mental illness is the feeling that you're a failure. It can arise as a result of relapses during recovery and other setbacks, and past experience with failure.

Amber

Amber was 23 and struggling with depression and cocaine addiction. She told me that her life was one big problem after another.

When Amber was 14 she dated a 17-year-old boy – her first boyfriend. He was popular and lived on the edge. He taught her to use drugs and was very controlling. If Amber wanted to go to the mall, to the movies or out to eat, she had to go with him. He believed that because she's beautiful, Amber would cheat on him. He told her that if she ever did, he would kill her. This dangerous boyfriend began to remove all that was good from her life. She no longer had friends, was using cocaine and alcohol, and was ruining her relationship with her family.

Amber's mom and dad wanted her to stay away from her boyfriend. They pointed out that she was failing in school, losing her friends and becoming a drug addict – all because of him. At 16, Amber made a bad choice. Her boyfriend convinced her to move in with him and stop talking to her parents. Things went from bad to worse. Amber spiraled out of control and nearly died.

At 18, Amber overdosed and fell into in a coma. Her family visited her and prayed that she would live – and change her life.

Amber survived and had a heart-to-heart talk with her parents. They demanded that she go to rehab and stay away from her boyfriend. Amber went to rehab and stayed away from him for three months. In a weak moment, she relapsed and reconnected with him.

Over the next six months Amber lost all that she had gained. She used cocaine daily and lived on the streets with her boyfriend. She almost died after another overdose. When her family asked me to help, I began to work with her. Amber told me that she had failed her parents and herself. She was upset over her relapse and her choice to rejoin her boyfriend.

I shared an important lesson with Amber: you must be willing to begin again. Even if you've made poor choices or failed in the past, you must be willing to change and start over again. We worked through many coaching sessions to help her break free from drugs and her boyfriend. The steps we took helped her to turn her life around.

Amber got a restraining order against her boyfriend and moved back into her parents' home. She went back to rehab and completed an outpatient program. She found hope in Narcotics Anonymous, where she met other women who were fighting addiction and rebuilding their lives.

A year has passed since I started working with Amber. She now has several friends who care about her and support her. They live sober and regularly attend meetings. Amber and her parents have a beautiful, healthy relationship. She plays tennis with her mom three times a week. She and her dad enjoy fishing and relaxing at her parents' lake house.

Amber is learning to make better relationship choices. She has decided to wait two years until she begins to date again. She has also agreed that she will consider her parents' opinion about her next relationship. Amber has made friends with men in recovery who are also rebuilding their lives. These days she is healthy, happy, drug-free and connected to those around her. It's been wonderful to watch this beautiful young woman turn her life around. She has many goals and plans for the rest of her life.

It took me a long time to realize that I had to begin again. During my struggles with mental illness there were times when I lost hope. A great doctor told me that I could only deal with today, and had to decide for myself whether to start my life again. Recovery meant taking baby steps and changing each aspect of my life. When I took those small steps, most areas of my life began to flourish. I began to accept my past and without being overwhelmed by the pain.

Evan

I once worked with a man in his forties named Evan. He'd lived a wild life, using and dealing drugs. Evan had hurt a lot of people and had been in and out of jail. When I met him, he'd been sober for several years.

Evan told me that his past did not define him. There was no way to change his history. If he chose to let them, those experiences could cause him to give up on himself. Evan says that he believes he has the rest of his life to be productive and helpful in the world.

Evan is a frequent speaker at AA meetings. He also works as a manager at a fruit store. The customers love his positive attitude, funny stories and kindness. The job has been perfect for him because he loves helping others. His great work ethic has enabled him to move from a cashier's job to manager.

Evan dreams of one day owning a health food store. He deposits $50 from every paycheck into a savings account, saving $1,400 so far. Evan has put together a business plan: when he saves $11,000 he'll open his new business. He taught me how important it is to try again and believe in yourself. He is a shining example of a man who never gives up.

I believe that all of us are born to overcome our problems. If God gave each of us free will, then it is up to us to choose. When you choose change, you can shift your thinking. You find that you're able to slowly change your behaviors, habits and even addictions. You might learn that your potential is remarkable.

I know many people in recovery who have contributed to their communities. What would happen if all of us overcame our addictions and went on to live our lives in healthy and constructive ways? I believe that our world would become a place of hope, healing and joy. When you make positive changes in your life you make the whole world a better place. Your regained health enables those who love you to feel confidence in you and be proud that you have moved forward.

Here's a tool that can help you with letting go. Sit somewhere quiet and ask God to take away your past. Tell God that you're sorry, and are willing to do the work necessary to change. Ask to be set free from the darkness and gloom of your addiction. You have the power to surrender and accept God's help.

During hard times, the only way to go on is with God's help. When I'm struggling, I know that drugs or alcohol will not help me. They'll only take the pain away for a short time, then it will come back much worse than before. This is the repetitive cycle of addiction. But love of God will never take you to a bad place. It will inspire, motivate, and encourage you to start your life again.

I haven't shared this often, but God is my best friend. When I have a problem, or feel lonely or lost, I ask for God's help. I talk to God often, asking for advice and assistance. God took the darkest pain of my mental illness and showed me how to use it to help others. God took the heartbreak of losing my only brother and used it to make me stronger. I was angry when Adam died, but the loss has enabled me to share powerful lessons about addiction. It also taught me how valuable life is, and that drugs can take everything from us.

When I lost my brother, part of me wanted to die, to give up and sink into addiction. Some of my family members chose to escape their feelings through alcohol and other drugs. During my brother's memorial service, many of them drank. I chose not to do so, so I had to confront my raw feelings. My only help came from God and my family. God gave me the courage to press on and begin again. I'm stronger and healthier today because I made the right choices.

I'm using my brother's death to share lessons with those who are willing to turn their lives around. I wish he didn't die, that he would have changed his life instead. God has helped me to accept that this wasn't possible, and so I must begin again. I recently found a beautiful journal that my brother kept during one of his stints in rehab. He wrote about how much he loved me and was proud of the person that I had become. Adam wrote that he was happy that I'd overcome my mental illness and was helping others. He also saved a note that I'd written to him. In it, I told him how much I loved him and how proud I was of him. I told him that I believed in him, loved him and knew he could do anything.

I wrote that note before he became addicted and lost his life. I'm happy he knew how much I cared about him. Even though he is dead, God allows me to talk to his spirit. I feel connected to him and will never let go of my love for him. He had a beautiful soul, and led a life of adventure.

I thank God for allowing me to start again. I've seen the darkness fade and be replaced by hope, light, love and a new beginning. I ask God to do the same in your life. My brother would be happy that I'm sharing his life to help others. He'd be honored if you'd get off drugs and stay drug free.

6: Fear

We've all faced fear. We might feel nervous about being different, angering others or failing. Many people become addicted because of fear. It's more comfortable to feel safe than to face the unknown.

Wally

Wally was a kind man. He was 48 and had a long history of alcohol addiction. We spoke about that history, and about how he dealt with fear by drinking.

Wally's fears range from being nervous around others and being a disappointment to his wife, to failing in his business. He told me that when he was a child, he felt happy only when everyone he loved was pleased with him. In trying to be perfect in their eyes, he lost himself. Together, we looked into who he really is.

Wally told me that he loves to dance, go to concerts, travel, write plays and act in playful way. I asked him how often he was true to himself, involved in these activities. He admitted that, at the time we spoke, it was close to never.

He cried as he admitted to me that his life was no longer fun. He was afraid that his marriage wasn't working, his job left him feeling empty and his drinking might have damaged his liver.

We talked about what he could do. I told him that it would be hard for him to change. He might "upset the applecart," so others would not be pleased with him. But his only other option was to keep doing the same things. If he continued to live the same way as he had been, he'd die from liver failure. Even worse, he would die unhappy and unfulfilled. I asked him how that would feel.

Wally answered that he agreed with me. He said that he had to face his fears and that his current path was a dead end. We agreed that he suffers from depression, in addition to his alcohol addiction.

Over the next several months Wally began to face his problems. He entered couples counseling with his wife to help them work through their marital difficulties. They decided to make the adjustments necessary for them to stay together. Those changes included Wally being able to make and maintain his own friendships, to travel and to attend concerts. He also began to rebuild his sex life. He and his wife went from making love once a month to once a week. He no longer used porn as a substitute for the love he needed from his wife.

Wally took a medical leave from his job, entered rehab, and spent three months there to stop drinking. During that time he met others who, like him, live with addiction. He learned that his story was a common one, and that many other "pleasers" end up in recovery.

After leaving rehab, Wally returned to work. He decided to build a boat, depositing part of his salary each week in a boat fund. He eventually built a large boat. Every Sunday he and his two best friends would attend concerts, listening to the music he loves.

Many people believe that confronting their fears is too difficult, so they don't even try. I've learned that fear is not real. We create it so that we don't have to change. Many of us are scared to be who we really are.

I used to have many fears. Here's one: what if I'm not good enough or don't please those around me? I eventually learned that I had to face fear to become the person I am. I built my own business, helping those with mental illness and addiction. I travel the world, educating and teaching. I've written (and continue to write) bestselling books. I'm rich – monetarily, and in happiness. It took me until age 35 to accept myself. Now I refuse to do anything that my heart is not in. My life is fun and free. I've accepted the adventures that I've had and can't wait to begin the beautiful journeys ahead.

Mali

I met a young woman named Mali. She was born in South Carolina and came from a long line of textile business owners. Her dad was rich and he loved Mali very much. He demanded that she attend a top college and marry a rich man. Mali finished school and was pushed into dating someone her parents thought was right for her. She was unhappy, and started using opiates to escape the situation. This went on for two years, until she overdosed.

Mali went through rehab and came out realizing that she needed to change. She moved to Australia and attended art school. While there, she met a handsome young sculptor named Lyle. He was also a former opiate abuser. They fell in love and backpacked throughout Europe. Mali and Lyle got married, but told her parents afterwards. She felt that she didn't need their approval because her life belongs to her. She now leads a simple, happy life filled with art, friends and true love.

I encourage you to face your fears. Your best chance to be happy is to learn what you want to do with your life. You'll be better able to end your addictions if you're satisfied and fulfilled. Life is short: it's up to you to take action now.

If you face up to your fears, who knows what you might accomplish? You may live the life you've dreamed about. When you leave fear behind, you can begin to travel a road to fulfillment. If you don't face your fears, you'll never be able to make that journey. You owe it to yourself to change.

Fear can make some experiences seem worse than they are. I recently moved to Florida and love being near my mom, dad, sister, father-in-law and brother-in-law. But my wife has not been happy there and wants to leave.

I applied for admission to several summer educational programs for new business owners. Admission is very competitive: as many as 300 people apply for only ten spots in each program. Those who are accepted spend several months sharpening their business skills, connecting with mentors and locating funding.

I knew that this would be a fun and enjoyable way for me to continue my growth. My wife was also excited to leave Florida for the summer while helping me to build my company. We were accepted into one of the best programs. I was thrilled, but also nervous about what my family would think about my wife and I leaving for 12 weeks. I was afraid that they might be angry, and that it would cause a huge fight. I recalled the feelings that were hurt when I left New York. It was as if I was making a choice between personal, professional goals and staying close to my parents. I love being close to my family. If we had healthy boundaries, we could enjoy the bond we share.

As summer approached I began to feel nervous. Would my parents be sad or angry if we left for the summer? All of us are still somewhat fragile emotionally following the deaths of my brother and grandmother and my other grandmother's stroke. Was I being selfish for wanting to attend this program? Do I only please my wife and not my family? I was upset about having to choose.

I spent a rainy Monday morning with my mom. She was helpful, as always. She brought my daughter a bathing suit. Why? Because when I took my daughter to school that day, the whole class was in their swimming gear: my daughter had forgotten that they were going on a swimming trip. My mom went out in the rain so that my daughter would have a bathing suit. Her caring and sharing have helped me to become a better man.

After the bathing suit problem was solved, my mother and I talked about what was going on in each other's lives. I wasn't ready to tell her about leaving Florida to attend the program because of FEAR. I was worried that I'd hurt her, which would hurt me. But when we finally addressed the subject, she said that it was fine with her if we went away for the summer. She'd visit us and would be happy to spend whatever time she could with us. She asked me if this was all that was going on. When I asked what she meant she became emotional. She'd been afraid that we were moving to California and were going to be gone for good!

Both of us had been afraid to talk about our fears, but when we faced them we realized that we had nothing to worry about. My wife and I decided to leave for the summer, then come back and build a better business. My mom can help me with my business whenever she wants to. *Her* fears were not even close to reality. *My* fears were a figment of my imagination. I've learned that it's better to be honest and open and to move forward. Sometimes your biggest fear is not a big deal after all.

Brad

Brad was a 30-year-old opiate addict. He was in rehab, consumed by fear. During the time when he abused drugs he had stolen from his grandmother, taking her wedding ring, her collection of gold jewelry, and even her television. Brad was ashamed at what he'd done. He cried in my office, overwhelmed by guilt and fear. He felt worthless because of the stealing he'd done.

I asked Brad how much his grandma loved him. He said that she considered him to be her best friend and would do anything for him. I pointed out that, by becoming sober, he had saved his life. Wouldn't his grandma be happy that he's going to survive? But he was still afraid of how she might react when he told her what he'd done.

Brad and I talked about the 12 steps in AA and NA. One of the most important steps is apologizing to those whom you have hurt during your addiction. He realized that he had to talk to his grandma. When she came to see him on visiting day she was overjoyed that his eyes were clear and he was healthier. During that visit Brad cried as he told her about his stealing. His grandma, Ruthie, began to cry as she listened. She said that she knew he had stolen from her, but would trade all of the gold in the world to have him alive and healthy. Ruthie forgave him and they hugged. She was thrilled that her Brad was going to make it, and Brad was relieved that his grandma (and best friend) forgave him. It was as if a thousand-pound boulder had been lifted off his chest. He became calmer, learned to forgive himself and was ready to move on.

Brad remained sober. He started helping others who needed and wanted to make changes in their lives. I watched him work with a sick addict who had a panic attack. Brad prayed for him and helped him through that tough time. I know he'll continue to make progress. His time of fear and depression is over, and he's ready to be the wonderful human being he's capable of being. I've seen the light come back into his eyes as he's released the darkness of fear. When he overcame his fear, he started on his way towards fulfilling his destiny.

If you're living with fear, NOW is the time to face it. Fear is a black hole in our minds and hearts. Face it, and you can move on. We've all made poor choices. I've apologized to many people whom I've hurt when I was suffering from mental illness. I believe that most of them have forgiven me and have been willing to put it behind us. You can move forward and stop the hurt inside you. You can learn to let go of fear and embrace your true self.

Blake LeVine

7: Developing a Positive Attitude

When I was a boy I had a negative attitude. I focused on what was wrong, and thought about my problems all the time. This enabled me to avoid having to be happy. I was so nervous that it was hard for me to feel okay.

As I grew up, I learned that attitude was everything. For years I worked to surround myself with inspiration and hope. One of the keys to doing this successfully was to repeat affirmations. When I woke up in a bad mood I'd say "I feel terrific, wonderful and healthy." In the beginning it seemed phony, but after months of practice I began to believe it.

I noticed that when I was positive, I felt more alive. Nowadays I'm almost always happy. I've learned that I don't have to let situations determine my emotions.

It all began with traffic. My dad would always get angry whenever we got stuck in a traffic jam. He'd yell, hit the steering wheel and call himself stupid for getting stuck! When I started driving I did the same things, but then I realized that I was making myself uncomfortable for however long I was stuck in traffic. I decided that I wasn't going to let traffic jams do that to me. I listened to music, laughed, thought of creative ideas and had fun whenever I got stuck. Now I don't care if I get caught in it (well, not much). I allow myself extra traveling time when I have an appointment and, if I run into traffic, I don't worry about being late.

As I became a happier person I faced situations that were more difficult to deal with than traffic jams. They included my brother's death due to a heroin overdose, my grandmother's death and my other grandma's stroke. Some might say that it was "o.k." for me to be depressed in these situations. They'd understand if I fell into addiction as a result. I could easily tell myself that the loss of loved ones gives me a "reason" to be unhappy. But I chose to not to give up feeling good.

Am I sad about losing my only brother? More than I know how to tell you. I miss him and would do anything to have him back. But I know that Adam would want me to keep living a good life. It would hurt his soul if I gave up because he's no longer here. The best way I can honor him is to press forward and be happy.

Since Adam died I've become closer to my family. I no longer fear each new day – instead I see it as a special gift. I know that I won't always be here and that my life should be as prosperous and joyous as I can make it. My attitude impacts those around me. By living this way, I help my family heal.

Xavier

Xavier was depressed and addicted to alcohol. He told me that life had beaten him down. His mother died when he was 12 and his dad was a cocaine dealer. He lived with his grandparents. His poppy and nanny made him feel comfortable and safe.

When Xavier was 15 his grandparents both died within a year of each other. He was forced to live with an aunt in Oklahoma. He was beaten at school, ridiculed, and completely isolated. He drank to escape. When we met he was 23 and struggling. He didn't want to live, and his addiction was consuming him. As we talked, he began to cry.

Xavier felt that God had taken everything away from him. I told him that he was right: it wasn't his fault that he'd lost his parents and grandparents. I asked him an important question: "What would your mom and grandparents want if they were alive?" He perked up and said "They would want me to work – to pursue my career as an auto mechanic and get married." I told him that if he stopped drinking he could do it.

Xavier and I also spoke about his conversations with himself. He told himself that he was a failure, worthless and a screw-up. I told him that he needed to change the tone of that conversation. Together, we identified things about him that were positive: he's strong, a survivor, good at fixing cars, and kind to animals.

Over the next several years Xavier changed his way of living. He woke up each morning thanking God for giving him another day. His conversation with himself became a positive one: He repeated his affirmations and began to believe that he is a good man. Xavier also became a Christian and went to church every day. He found hope among the other church members and made some wonderful friends. He became an optimistic and joyous human being.

Xavier built his own auto repair shop, specializing in foreign cars. He met a woman and fell in love. Eventually, they were married. Xavier and I talked about how proud his family would be of him. He says that he knows his family in heaven watches over him. If you met Xavier today you wouldn't suspect that he'd been through so much pain and sorrow. He is a wonderful member of his community who mentors troubled youth and gives of his life in many other ways.

There are many examples of people who overcame difficulties and turned their lives around. Thomas Edison created some of the most remarkable inventions in history. Did you know that he was fired from his job and, at one time, was almost penniless? Beethoven created music that continues to touch our world. How many know that he lost his hearing – and kept on composing? You may not have heard of Olaudah Equiano. As a boy he was brought to America as a slave. He eventually gained his freedom and wrote a book about his life. It influenced opinion in Britain and played a major part in ending slavery.

What would happen if you turned your life around? Is there something you could contribute to our world? The common element in all of these lives is a determination to develop and maintain a positive attitude, even during severe challenges.

Our attitudes impact everything in our lives. I like to tell people about a remarkable turning point in my life. When I was a teenager I went on a ski vacation with one of my best friends, Harrison. We went to Beaver Creek, Colorado, an area that features beautiful mountains covered in snow. During our week there we enjoyed snowmobiling and skiing. Once I went up to the top of a massive mountain with Harrison, who is an expert skier. I decided that it was more than I could handle and slid down the mountain on my butt. I didn't go back up. Instead, I sat at a fire pit, relaxing and enjoying the view. A young man, about my age, also sat at the fire. We started to talk and became friends.

I would never have guessed that this young man was a billionaire! He was down to earth and dressed simply. He told me that his grandfather was the Prime Minister of Greece. We were both almost 18, but our lives would become much different when we reached our next birthday. When his day came, he would inherit a fortune. He planned to buy a boat and travel the world. I told him about my many adventures and he seemed impressed. He asked me to come with him to meet his mom.

I'll never forget my visit to the first-class hotel attached to the mountain. We went to the penthouse – his family had reserved the entire floor, almost 18 rooms. When I met his mom I expected her to tell me that her life was perfect. She was rich, beautiful and had enough money to buy whatever she might want.

I told her about my experiences meeting famous people and the adventures I'd had, but added that the best part of my life was that I was happy. She laughed and told me that this was impossible. She said that she knew the wealthiest people and all of them were miserable, including her. There was a man in the room, and I asked her if he was her husband. She again laughed and said she couldn't marry him because he had a low-level job in the government and, if they were married, she'd lose her title. None of it made sense to me. She had it all but was miserable. I realized then and there that money is not the key to happiness. Love, joy, and a positive attitude are more valuable. Success is in your heart, not in what you have.

I received another important lesson from a life coach, Randy Spelling. We were both around the same age, and had been around famous people since our youth. I hired Randy to help me. We did a weekly session, talking about life.

I thought that Randy's life must have been easy because his dad was the legendary producer, Aaron Spelling. While he was growing up he lived in The Manor, which is a mansion in Holmby

49

Hills, California. At one time it was listed for sale for $150 million.

As we worked together, Randy shared one of his most valuable lessons: you never should walk in someone else's shoes. Many have assumed, wrongly (like me), that his life had been easy. The truth is that he had to work hard to build his career. While doing so, he moved away from California to make his own way in life. He's a brilliant young man who found his path in helping others. It was great to meet another young man who had walked away from a privileged background and became known for helping others. I consider him to be a friend, and I'm honored to have had him teach and coach me towards positive change.

When Randy and I worked together I lived in a small apartment and money was tight. He helped me to envision a beautiful home and wealth. I called him a year later to tell him that I was living in a beautiful home in a great neighborhood, surrounded by terrific people. I was enjoying an abundance of happiness and was doing well financially. Randy's teaching played a big part in making these goals become real.

We all need someone who will uplift, motivate and encourage us. Don't battle through negative feelings and emotions on your own. I've put together a team of caring professionals to help you work through your difficulties. We offer you a free counseling session to get you started. Visit our website, http://www.bipolaronline.com, to learn more about our offer.

You may find that the effort it takes to be positive will be the best investment you ever make. When you see someone who is rich or famous – but who is also sad – it should remind you that possessions are not true wealth. Some of the homeless New

Yorkers with whom I've worked are happier than some of the richest and most famous people. I'm not asking you to live with nothing, but you are allowed to be happy. You must believe in yourself and always press forward.

NOW is a great time to start working on who you are. You have the ability to progress and stay positive. It may be a long road, but it is never too late to start. Don't give up on living a happier life.

Many people who have addictions lose their positive attitude. If you fall too far into addiction, you may always see your life as falling apart. Many who suffer from mental illness are also afraid to choose happiness. When your experiences have been negative, it's easy to be upset or to feel lost. When you begin to rebuild your life, you give yourself a chance to become the person you truly are. I've learned to be calmer, kinder and more relaxed, and to live in a peaceful way. I know I have more work to do – there's always more work to do – but I'm grateful to be on my peaceful journey.

8: Embracing Change

When you've lived with the darkness and pain of addiction it's hard to accept the challenge to change. But the only way you can survive and rebuild is to change. Even the most stable situations eventually change. It's part of our evolution as humans to continually adapt, grow and discover new ways to survive. One of the most useful survival tools is to realize – and accept – that when things change, you can adapt and live your life in a new way.

Katrina

Katrina was only 21 but had already lived through a lot of drama. Her dad was a cocaine addict who had left his family many years earlier. Her mom was a wonderful woman, but she did not have the patience to help Katrina with all of the feelings and issues she was dealing with. Katrina lost contact with her brother when he moved away at age 15.

Katrina suffered from severe mental health difficulties since her youth. It began with acting out in school and fighting with other kids. She was thrown out of high school for beating a girl with a bat. Her emotions were strong and were never properly addressed. She refused to take medication. Her life was scary.

Katrina was placed in a hospital/school for girls with mental health problems. She was mean and defiant, even in this controlled setting. After fighting the system throughout the time she was there, she was released on her 18th birthday. All she'd known in her life was pain and trouble.

Katrina was sad and lonely, but started finding happiness in getting high. She began with marijuana but quickly moved on to crystal meth. Katrina had never been addicted to a serious drug and was no longer treating her mental health. Her life was so difficult that she hoped she would die. Death seemed easier than seeking help and starting over.

Katrina's wish was granted: she overdosed, but was resuscitated in time so she survived. When her mom came to visit her, Katrina told her how much pain and hurt she felt.

Over the next two years she made some small changes. She began seeing a psychiatrist to help her deal with her moods. She found a combination of anti-psychotic and mood-stabilizing drugs that helped her stabilize her life. Katrina also began to seek help for her addiction. She spent a year going to a treatment center to learn how to stay away from drugs.

Working together, Katrina and I set goals and made changes. We discovered that, along with all of the rest, Katrina was a talented singer. She had an amazing voice and raw charisma. Katrina decided that she wanted to be a wedding and event singer. Through an ad she placed on craigslist.org she found three other musicians to work with her. Within a month, Katrina had some business cards printed and developed a pricing schedule. Within a year, business was booming.

Katrina feels pure exhilaration when she sings at events. She loves watching the eyes of a happy couple and being a part of their special day. Her business has been successful, providing her with regular work.

Katrina was proud that she found the courage to change her life. The angry, intense and miserable girl was replaced by a smart, happy, successful young woman. Her story demonstrates that all of us have the potential to accomplish great things if we're willing to change.

Willingness to change has enabled me to harness my powers to achieve. I used to be lazy, unwilling to put in a full effort. I was upset with myself because I knew that I wasn't using my gifts. As I began to overcome my resistance I realized that I love to work! It's fun to wake up each day and be creative and productive. On a rare day when I sleep in, I sometimes regret that I haven't gotten up and made use of my time. My brother's death continues to teach me that it's necessary to use your days wisely. We never know how much time is left or when it will end.

Wouldn't it be great to end your addiction and become mentally stable? What if YOUR change enabled you to become what God wants you to be? Take the steps to turn your life around. This means no more excuses or justifying your negative behavior. It's up to you to make it happen. Each of us are on our own path. Your family, friends and coach can't change you. You must allow yourself to evolve and grow.

Duke

Duke had plenty of self-esteem. When he was in high school, everyone in his small town knew about Duke and his wild escapades. He was the undisputed life of the party, consuming fishbowls full of liquor. Duke thought that his lifestyle was working for him: He was cool, had a lot of friends and woman adored him. Duke had a lot of sex. The girls he hooked up with were just as intoxicated as he was.

Duke liked to watch rap videos. They showed him people who lived the same fast life as he did: beautiful women, drugs, sex and parties. Duke didn't see any reason why the party should ever end, but his parents worried that eventually he'd fall apart.

Things started to go bad during his junior year. He'd been a "B" student, but now he couldn't seem to wake up in the morning and started cutting classes. Duke barely completed the 11th grade and wanted to drop out. During senior year, he started using harder drugs, including cocaine, "molly" (MDMA) and eventually heroin. He watched as his friends moved on to college. Duke became depressed and was lost in his addiction. He started injecting heroin instead of just snorting it. He no longer was the life of the party, just another sad drug addict.

Duke still had a few friends. Together, they'd get high. They began breaking into cars to get money for drugs. They were arrested when they took a small amount of money (change) from a car that belonged to an undercover detective. Duke received a long jail sentence, but got a lucky break during a court appearance.

The judge told Duke that he knew he was an addict. He said that his daughter (who knew about Duke) had told him so, but that he could see it for himself in Duke's bloodshot eyes. As an alternative to jail, the judge offered to remand Duke to a one-year treatment center. If he stayed sober, he would not be charged with a felony. It was up to Duke whether to go to jail or choose to be sober. He decided that his fast life was over and accepted the deal. He asked God for help.

Instead of being the life of the party, Duke became the life of rehab. He made friends, opening up to them and releasing his emotions. He organized a baseball game and found hope in the other men in recovery. Duke chose to change and to face his fears. He realized that he didn't lose his gift – being able to connect with people – when he stopped using drugs.

While he was in rehab, Duke decided to become a car salesman. He knew that his love of cars and driving would help him in this work. By the time he completed his year in rehab and went back before the judge, Duke was fully alive, hopeful, energetic and at peace. The judge was impressed by the glowing report that the rehab facility gave him, and by what he saw. Duke had changed: he was ready and willing to live the life he was capable of living.

Duke became the general manager of a local Honda dealership. He was so talented that the dealership became one of the top-ranked in sales for four years in a row. He married a beautiful woman who is also in recovery. They have two children and live a life of happiness and joy. Duke still socializes, but now he does it without getting high. He's embraced the fact that fun does not mean drugs and alcohol. He takes his kids boating, fishing and whitewater rafting. Duke learned that his spark – the thing that draws people to him – burns brighter when he stays away from drugs and alcohol.

Sometimes we have to walk away from our past in order to change. This might mean walking away from friends and family members. It doesn't mean that you're disloyal if you decide that some of the people in your life are toxic. When you become sober, you must decide for yourself who will be involved in your new life. Friends who get high each day won't support you in sobriety. When you attend Alcoholics Anonymous or Narcotics Anonymous meetings, you'll find people who live free from drugs and alcohol. Find the best group of friends to associate with. That group can include family members and friends, but limit contact to an occasional visit if they stir up too many difficult emotions. It's hard to walk away from what you've always known, but sometimes you must.

Many addicts associate with the same people – and have the same problems – for years. It's more comfortable for them to do this than to travel the hard road of recovery. But their approach is a dead end, and it will always be a dead end. The only way to succeed is to travel the path that leads to love, light and healing – no matter how difficult it may be. You wouldn't be reading these words if you didn't need to change. It's going to take a lot of courage for you to do the work you know you have to do. The good news is that you only have to take one small step to begin. This small step leads to more, and eventually you'll find yourself walking steadily on the right path.

You only need to deal with today. Are you ready to set new goals? Are you willing to give up the dysfunction that has stopped you from moving forward? What will it take for you to be willing to live in a healthy way? These are questions that you must answer for yourself. Take a moment and think about them. You might find that you know the right answers and are ready to change.

9: The Longer Road

Why do we want fast food? How come there are so many websites offering instant answers? Is it because we have no time, or that we want life-on-demand? I've considered these questions often, with respect to my own life. For years I wanted everything NOW. This included a successful career and lots of money. A pattern developed: I wanted something, tried to get it, then gave up when it didn't come to me as quickly as I desired. As I took on more responsibilities, I became more frustrated. How could I wait for success while I had a wife and two children to support? If it was going to take a year, but I only had enough money for a month, how could I be patient? I eventually achieved the success that I wanted, but first I had to accept slower travel on a longer road.

It took me a long time to earn my degree in social work. It took even longer to build a practice and develop the tools to be successful. I had to learn how to promote my services, build websites, network with clients, manage finances – and be patient. I waited two years for my first book to be purchased by a major publisher. I wanted it to be published as soon as I finished writing it! I needed money, and was hoping that it would provide me with a lot of it.

Instead, I learned that the true value of my book was in helping me share my knowledge, and to make people aware of my coaching practice. I traveled throughout California promoting it. I spent thousands of hours creating web pages to tell people my story. I created hundreds of videos, encouraging others to learn about it.

That was my first book. I'm writing this one with a much healthier attitude. I know that I have to be patient and accept that it will be done – and in the hands of those who need it – when all of the work necessary to put it there is finished. I've decided that I'll release it myself. This will enable me to increase my publishing knowledge, and I'll benefit financially over the years it will continue to sell (and I'm confident that it will). I'm not writing this book for instant gratification. I'm writing it to share valuable lessons and to encourage you to find hope. My brother would be pleased that, by sharing his life, I'll help others who struggle with addiction.

The longer road is often so obvious that we miss it. We're so stuck in NOW that we can't wait patiently. We're afraid we'll be late.

I went to breakfast with my six year old daughter Tyler. She had just finished school for the year and my wife was working all day. I knew that keeping Tyler active would be a good way to help her handle the transition of not being in school.

We woke up early and went to her favorite breakfast place – the International House of Pancakes. Tyler had eggs, bacon and pancakes. I wanted to eat healthier, so I had my morning cup of coffee at the restaurant and decided to eat breakfast at home.

When we got back I had fruit and whole grain cereal. I ate what was good for me and saved money. I had to wait an extra hour to eat, but it was worth it. I'm glad that I avoided the heavy pancakes and waffles that I thought about having. I do, once in a while, enjoy these foods, but I didn't want to begin the summer by making them an everyday habit.

Jan

Jan was a terrific client who seemed to have it all. He had stopped drinking, was happily married and owned a big company that helped other businesses obtain loans. I asked him what lessons he had learned to achieve so many of his goals.

Jan told me that when he was younger he wanted everything instantly. When he decided that he wanted the fastest bike, he got a newspaper route. When he was older and wanted a nice car, he started an Amazon business. He got the bike and car he wanted, but not as quickly as he had hoped.

It took him three years to save enough money to buy his first Ford Mustang. He watched as other friends in his wealthy town got the cars they wanted – given to them on their 17th birthdays. On his 17th birthday, Jan got his driver's license, but only had half of the money he needed to buy the car he dreamed about. His could either buy a cheaper car or be patient. Jan chose to keep working and saving, and one year later he had enough.

Jan says he learned that some things are worth the wait. When he set other goals – he wanted a plane and several homes – Jan had to work hard and save for many years. His early lessons taught him to never give up and eventually he got what he wanted. These days he is happy, wealthy – and patient. He doesn't lose hope when life takes time.

When I was a boy my dad gave me a small amount of money from his earnings. By the time I was 18, I had accumulated about $10,000. I told him that I wanted the money NOW, and that I was ready to handle it. This was during the internet boom of the 1990s. Each day many stocks shot up and it seemed as if anyone could make money.

I became a trader, using the money my dad gave me. My first trade went well: I made $500. I was happy and sure that I'd soon be seriously rich. The next day I bought a stock with a market order. This means that the stock would be purchased at its opening price, whatever that might be. I was excited and believed that I had a winner. It opened at $2.00 and I bought 4,000 shares (I thought it would open at 50 cents). My cost was $8,000. By the end of the trading day it was worth $2,000. Within one week it was worth $1,000. I was devastated. I'd lost $7,000 of the money I had worked years to save.

I almost didn't tell my dad. When I did, he was very angry. I learned (the hard way) that a desire for quick riches can lead you to lose much (or all) of what you have.

When I was a little older I decided to invest in real estate. One investment, in an apartment, turned out to be a ten-year road. I had to deal with a fire in the building, difficult tenants, and I even went through a time when I owed the bank money. I persisted through all of it and eventually sold the apartment. The money I earned enabled me to pay off my college student loan in full. I also bought several smaller investment properties with the money from sale. I created long-term income by doing some long-term thinking. It's helped me to become financially secure.

You might see some of yourself in these experiences. Have there been times when you chose quick-and-easy instead of slow-and-steady? What if you began to walk a slower and more achievable path? You might decide to live in a way that gives you the best chance at success.

Many people have achieved wonderful goals by taking their time. "Rome was not built in a day." Almost anything worth doing will take longer than you anticipate. I've found that when you let go and do the daily work you'll develop a winning attitude. It's common to find more peace on the longer, slower road. When you're rushed and pushed you don't have time to plan and win.

Irene

Irene was a talented woman who felt intense pressure to achieve. When she was in her 20s she became addicted to drinking and suffered a breakdown. Her high level of inner pressure and constant rushing around fueled her addiction. She didn't take care of herself.

She knew it had to stop. I asked Irene how much she did in an average day. She told me that she often started her day with a list of 50 goals that she wanted to accomplish before it was over. She worked from 7am to 11pm to do so. When she failed to finish her list she'd cry. She felt like a loser and drank each night. It was clear that she was putting too much pressure on herself. I asked her where was the time for fun, joy and peace in her schedule? Why did she always need to do so much?

Irene admitted that she was trying to escape from life. She was unhappy and lonely. She always put herself down and didn't feel worthy of love. She used constant work to cover up how she really felt.

We began a program to help her accept herself. She started to focus on the good in her life. She also forgave her first love, who broke her heart. The pain from this relationship had prevented her from enjoying her life.

Irene changed some of her habits. She began to work only eight hours a day and to limit herself to ten goals. This enabled her to find time each night to exercise using a Yoga video. She took a bath for 30 minutes to help her to slow down and relax. She enjoyed using bubble bath and playing Sarah McLachlan CDs. Irene traveled to Paris for three weeks. She'd always wanted to see that beautiful city. As she released the pressure, she began to enjoy a calmer, slower life.

There's no need to rush through life, but the pressure we put on ourselves sometimes traps us into doing so. You can be productive without entering a rat race. The long-term success we all want is achieved by those who make slow, steady progress. It's easier to walk at a pace you can handle than to run at a speed you can't maintain.

When you're young, it's hard to imagine yourself at 60 or 70. But many, probably most, of us will reach such an age. What if, over the course of many years, you accomplished your goals? Here are some numbers to illustrate what I mean. If you accomplish 50 goals a day you'll achieve 250 in a five-day period (a standard work week). But when you burn out, that's the end of goal-achievement for you. On the other hand, if you accomplish 10 goals per day for a five-day week, that's 50 goals a week and over 2,500 per year. Do that for 20 years and you will have achieved 50,000 goals. What would your life be like if you slowly, steadily achieved 50,000 goals?

How about if you saved $10 a day? That's $50,000 after 20 years. If over the next twenty years you save $100 a day you'll end up with $500,000! How much money have you wasted on drugs or alcohol? Did you find $10 a day to spend on your addiction? What would happen if you slowly, steadily saved money or worked on goals? This is why people like Warren Buffett and Bill Gates have enormous wealth. They've taken the path of slow-and-steady. You might be the next billionaire if you develop your ability to slowly and steadily work on your goals. If you do so, you'll also simplify your life.

It took me a long time to develop these habits. I continue to do my best to live this way day-to-day. I used to buy lottery tickets hoping for a "big win." I was wasting about $50 a week on it. I usually lost, or at most won $4. I decided to save that $50 a week instead. After three months, I had over $600. I used the money in some wonderful ways. I celebrated a birthday with a beautiful dinner with my wife. I bought a new computer to help me make videos and grow my business. I love my new computer and use it every day. Among other things, I've used it to sell old items on Ebay. I've earned back the money I spent on my computer by using it in this way. Instead of throwing money away I've used it for things that I enjoy.

I still want to win the lottery. The difference is that I know that I can guarantee a "big win" for myself over a long period of time, using the slow-and-steady approach.

If I continue to grow my income, I'll be able to save $300 a week. That's $15,000 a year. With that amount I can buy an apartment or a small house each year. Over 30 years I'll own 30 homes with no mortgages, all producing rental income. I expect the homes to be valued at over $5 million.

To me, this sounds like winning the lottery, except that the odds of it happening are close to 1:1. The odds of winning the Powerball jackpot in the United States are currently 1 in

175,223,510.00. Which would YOU choose? Many people believe it would be more fun to win Powerball, and I agree that it would be pretty cool to have my picture taken next to a giant check. But I've learned that knowing that I've built long-term wealth at low risk is the way to greater peace of mind.

10: Your Inner Fire

I've always had hobbies, interests and passions. When I had to deal with my mental illness and breakdown, all of them vanished. My focus was on survival and, later, trying to live outside of a hospital. Pursuing my passions was a minor concern, if that. As I rebuilt my life, my attention was focused on finding the right doctors and therapies, and understanding why things had happened to me. I was unable to attend school, maintain friendships, date or do much of anything. Thoughts of writing a book, movie or play, or of traveling, were the furthest things from my mind.

As I began to recover, things changed. I remembered how I'd enjoyed pursuing my passions. I worried that maybe my inner fire had gone out and might not be relit. Sometimes I thought that my medication dulled me, and that I wouldn't be able to achieve anything as long as I was on it.

While attending college, I started to believe that my inner fire hadn't gone out after all. I had always enjoyed meeting notable people, so I started a public access television show, interviewing celebrities at different events in New York City. I was nervous at first, but found that I was good at speaking to famous people and asked them good questions. Also, I enjoyed building relationships with publicists and developing a good reputation as a reliable interviewer.

I interviewed Walter Cronkite, Justin Timberlake, Katie Couric, Barbara Walters, Sue Simmons, Ben Affleck, Matt Damon, James Taylor, and many other big names. The night of September 10, 2001 was a big one for me. I was in the reporter line during a benefit for Michael Jackson. I interviewed the

Jackson family, Beyonce' Knowles, Slash (from Guns N' Roses) and many others.

I was still in New York the next day, September 11, when the World Trade Center was destroyed. This event and its aftermath inspired me to use my gifts to help others. I enrolled in a graduate program, studying Social Work, and began to feel my inner fire burning again – as a desire to help others.

That inner fire of mine has continued to burn as I've shared my life lessons in a number of ways, including several books and many educational talks. I feel free and fully alive when I share my story and help others who struggle to improve their lives. I no longer feel dull – I'm passionate about the inner fire in my life. I've learned it's necessary for us to pursue our passions in a manageable way. Many of those who suffer from addictions and mental illness have great potential. If you do what you love in a structured way, you're likely to see results that express your inner joy.

Gil

Gil suffered from cocaine addiction and bipolar disorder. After years of struggling to stay away from cocaine while trying to function mentally, he found the right combination of medications and began to attend NA meetings. He also attended meetings at The National Alliance on Mental Illness and their local support group. When we started working together he was doing well – on paper. He had a job, friends and had stayed away from coke for a while. The problem, he told me, was that he was bored. He felt as if something was missing from his life.

We began to examine his life history. Gil told me that he had a huge interest in sports. He loved to watch, attend games and even play football. He'd stopped playing several years earlier because of a back injury. Gil felt that his childhood dream of being a football star was far behind him.

Together, we came up with some great ways for him to be involved with the game he loved. Gil joined a league of touch football players. They played for three hours every Sunday. He also became a coach for a team in the local pee wee league. He said that these activities relit his inner fire and helped him to add excitement to his life. He believes that they are a positive release for his energies.

Julie

Julie was a beautiful woman who fell into addiction by accident. She was never a good student, so she left school and worked as a waitress at a local Italian restaurant. She loved working there, making friends with coworkers and enjoying the fast pace. After working there for three years she met Leo, a handsome young man with black hair. They began a relationship.

Julie didn't know that Leo was an opiate addict. When she found out, she looked past it because she loved him. Leo told her that he used opiates to relieve pain and that he didn't have a drug problem. When the local pill mills stopped supplying him he began to use heroin instead, but did not tell Julie.

During a night of drinking Leo used heroin and convinced Julie to try it. She became hooked and ended up battling addiction for a long time. It wasn't easy for her to leave Leo but she did. But after she left, he wouldn't leave her alone. They were both deep in their addictions. Julie's dad finally took her by plane to a rehab far from their home town.

Julie became drug free and committed to changing her life. She moved into a sober house. She decided not to work in a restaurant again because she was afraid to go back into the life she'd left behind, but she missed the fast-paced work environment.

As a result of our discussions about what kind of job would be good for her, Julie decided to become a teacher. That would certainly give her busy days, and would enable her to be around kids all of the time – something she was sure she'd like. Julie didn't want to go back to college, so she took a job at a preschool to get some hands-on experience. She loved it. The other teachers became her friends, and Julie loved the children she mentored.

This school had a very strict drug-use policy. Each teacher was drug-tested. Sometimes random tests were performed. The policy helped Julie to stay sober and ensured that the people she worked with were also drug-free. In the restaurant world, many of her coworkers drank, smoked pot and even used hard drugs. The restaurant turned a blind eye and did not seem to care about it. The school environment was healthier and safer for Julie. These days she's living her passions while chasing 15 or more five-year-olds around the classroom. I give a lot of credit to her for her patience and love of young people.

All of us have gifts and abilities. We must learn how to fulfill them by channeling our energy in productive, creative ways. Many who are addicted or suffer from mental illness are highly-creative people. They come alive when they are creating and engaged in activities that they love. It's hard for them work at jobs that don't provide an outlet for their joy.

It's important not to become a robot who feels no passion or joy. Find out what makes you feel most alive. What is it that you love and feel happy doing? If you could do whatever you want, what would you do? The answers to these questions help us to learn what we're passionate about.

Nick

Music can help us spiritually. Nick was in a 60-day rehab and was doing very well. He had stopped using opiates, made friends, helped clean the unit and seemed like a great person. But two weeks before he was to be released I was alerted that there was a problem: the staff had found him hiding an iPod in his bed. At this particular rehab they don't allow patients to have access to music. It was a major offense.

I took Nick into my office and asked him about the iPod. I wondered why a client who was doing so well would break one of the rules when he was close to being released. Nick told me that music was his passion. He was happiest when he could listed to his favorite bands: The Beatles, the Rolling Stones, Eric Clapton, Bob Dylan and Jeff Beck. He said that when he listened to music, he went to a better place. It was as if his soul resonated with the music. Nick said he was happy to be off drugs and he no longer wanted to use opiates, but he would not live without music.

I agreed that, in Nick's case, music was a tool for healing. After our conversation, I sometimes played music in the groups that I ran. I saw how happy it made the clients when I did. They were never happier than when the staff allowed them to bring in a guitar. They played songs, danced and generally lightened up. I held on to Nick's iPod after our talk, but eventually it was returned to him. He left the rehab and I'm sure that he's continuing to listen to his favorite tunes.

Music has also helped me to deal with my feelings and heal. When my brother died it left a void in my life. I listened to music to help me deal with the emptiness. I played songs that were about losing someone. Two of them, about the death of rapper Notorious BIG, helped me to reflect on my loss. I heard another great song on religious radio about the importance of forgiveness. It taught me to forgive my brother. It wasn't his fault that he was addicted. I shouldn't be angry at him because he had a medical problem. I made peace with his passing and forgave him.

I loved my little brother more than anything. I no longer have him with me, but I have music to express what I'm unable to say. In "The Message," Dr. Dre talks about his brother Tyree who died after being attacked. He raps about the plans he'd made with his brother, plans that would not be carried out. I relate to what this other doctor shared about what his brother meant to him. His words resonate deep in my soul.

Writing has enabled me to share my life lessons and to find energy and peace. It's one of the best outlets for feelings and one of the best ways to express one's gifts. Some books remain around for a long time. I believe that long after I'm dead what I've written will still be here. What if my writing helps someone two hundred years from now? How wonderful it is to use your words to inspire someone who is struggling, even if it's after you're gone.

My pain has been healed by the creative energy I've given to my inner fire. I could have remained alone with my pain but, by starting a new book, I invested my suffering in something that might do a lot of good.

Maybe your inner fire is different from mine, or from anybody's. Only you can truly know what you love to do. Find it and pursue it. You'll be happier and healthier when you do.

I hope you'll find the courage to believe in yourself. You might write a book, movie, play, article or song that uplifts many lives. I give you permission to be who you are —don't hide from your gifts. What a waste it would be to keep what God has given you hidden. Light up the world with the inner fire that burns inside you.

Blake LeVine

11: Sharing and Giving

Sometimes it seems as if we live in a world in which we only value things. This includes job status and other achievements, family and money. When you focus on *things* – to the exclusion of all else – you lose one of the keys to living a full life. I've met many people who were stuck in this way, trying to obtain things. They worried about not being able to obtain the things they wanted. But even when they got some of these things, they only wanted more. Sounds like addiction, doesn't it? Even if you score your drug today, it won't make you happy for very long. When it wears off, you'll be back to searching for your next fix.

I once fell into this pattern. I used to collect the autographs of famous people. As time passed, I began to think that fame – the kind they had – would fulfill me. It would take away my loneliness and help me to be loved. If I was a celebrity, everyone would care about me. So, for a long time, I tried to achieve my own version of fame.

What would it be like to be followed everywhere you go? To go on vacation and have photographers waiting in the bushes to take your picture? To pick up your child from school and have a pack of paparazzi waiting to photograph you – and your child? What would it be like to feel that you were always being watched and were never alone? It's a blessing that my childhood fantasies of being a famous star did not materialize. I thank God that he kept this from happening to me, even though I tried to achieve it.

The part of fame that has value is the part that you share with the world. I would not be as happy and fulfilled as I am if I hadn't learned to share the gifts I've received. I do this in a number of ways.

I love to go to Walmart and talk with the people who work there, brightening their day (and mine) in the process. When I go to a restaurant, I'm kind and friendly to the waiters and waitresses and thank them for their help. When I ask how their day is going, many are appreciative that I care enough to ask.

It was an honor to make friends with my daughter's teachers during this school year. Each day I told them how grateful I was for the kindness they showed her. I met a nice woman who babysits our neighbor's children. We spent 30 minutes discussing life and the joy of children. She told me that she hoped to have a big family with her new husband.

It's awesome to start the day by being kind or making a new friend. I've gone from watching my daughter by myself to making a new friend and having my daughter play with five other children down the block. Simple kindness can help you to rebuild your life following addiction and mental illness.

Andy

Andy was a smart, creative young man who battled depression and marijuana addiction. He ended up rehab after attempting to kill himself. Andy carried a lot of pain around with him. He didn't feel accepted. He was gay, and always looked and acted differently from others.

When we first met, Andy told me that he didn't think he deserved to live. It took him a long time to find the right anti-depressant medication and accept himself. Eventually, he developed a more positive attitude that included a focus on what's right about him. Andy is artistic, handsome, good with animals and very patient.

As he began his recovery, he looked for a way to give back. He volunteered at a shelter for abused dogs. Andy gave the animals the love and attention they deserved, but had not received. He worked there three days a week, walking, feeding, cuddling, and nurturing them. Many dogs thrived in his care and eventually found new homes.

Andy gave of his life and shared the gifts that God had given him. Helping those dogs led to a breakthrough for him. He no longer felt isolated, and contributed something worthwhile by using his talents. He made friends with the other volunteers, so he was no longer lonely. Today, he's happier than he's been in a long time and lives drug-free. You'd never know that he used to be severely depressed and addicted. Now he's an engaged and happy young man.

You may have been in some difficult situations during your life, but they haven't stopped you from giving of yourself. At least they shouldn't have. Each of us has special abilities that were given to us by God. When we share these abilities with others it helps us to open up to the possibility of healing.

One of the best parts of giving is how great it feels. In a way, sharing with others helps you as much as it helps them. Sometimes more. Human beings were created to connect with and help each other. Every living thing balances itself, and there's a place for all of them. Each plays a part in how the environment works. We need bees, plants, trees, sunlight and all of the rest.

How might you share your abilities to improve society? Small steps can be a big deal. When you talk to someone who tells you that he or she has no friends, how important is that discussion? When you love and care for a dog that has been abused and abandoned, how does the animal feel? If you are friendly towards someone who works at a difficult job, how much does it help them to know that you value their work?

Melissa

Melissa was a 19 year old girl who was abandoned by her dad and lived with her single mother. She learned at an early age to be self-sufficient. She had no time for fun. Her life was filled with responsibilities like paying the bills. As time went on, Melissa got tired. The pressure began to take its toll, and she started drinking beer. It started with one a night but quickly increased. She eventually drank 10-15 beers each night. Melissa knew that it was hurting her, so she questioned the way she was living, and looked for answers.

When we spoke, Melissa saw that she was filling a void with her addiction. She focused on ways that she could feel happier and less overwhelmed by responsibilities.

She began a project to help soldiers' families. She had an uncle who died in a war and had seen how hard it was on his wife and kids. The group that Melissa organized sent care packages to families who had a loved one who died in a battle. The packages were filled with books, drawings, food, and beautiful notes. She contacted local businesses, which donated items to include in the packages. The response from the families who received the packages was overwhelming. Many said that the gifts gave them new hope and helped them to realize that they were not forgotten.

Because she gave of herself, Melissa was no longer fixated on her own problems and responsibilities. Even though she'd added volunteer work to her schedule, she still had time for her job and for herself. Melissa was proud that she'd made a difference. Her volunteer work helped her to get through her addiction and to let go of the pressure she felt.

All of us are healthier when we use our talents to help others. Karma works: If you share your gifts, love will come back to you. I see kindness and warmth wherever I go, every day. When I'm friendly to people, they usually respond positively. Even when I meet a person who seems to be having a bad day they often cheer up when I speak to them. It doesn't bother me when someone says something mean to me. I know that it is often more about their struggles than anything I've said or done. I feel sorry for them, and know that they will have to work through their problems.

When I completed my graduate program in social work, I wanted to get some practical experience. I applied for a lot of jobs, but didn't hear from most of them. Finally I was offered an interview for a job at a non-profit agency in New York City, working with the homeless. I thought the job might be too hard and wasn't sure I should bother with the interview. But I went, and enjoyed meeting and speaking with the supervisor. It took four interviews for me to receive an offer, but I still wasn't sure I wanted the job. I finally accepted it, and began to work.

During the two years that I was with the agency, I saw a lot: homeless people talking to cars, using drugs, and fighting with each other. Sometimes I was scared when I approached them to offer food and services, but I also saw beauty during those years. I watched our homeless clients eat together in soup kitchens, holding hands as they gave thanks for their meals. They often shared their life lessons and knowledge with me.

Luigi was a painter who was also homeless. He was in his 50s and an addict. He got sober but couldn't afford an apartment in the city. Luigi told me that he'd seen many people get rich by investing in real estate. He also said that his family had lost a huge amount of money in the stock market. Luigi encouraged me to buy property, fix it up and re-sell it. He said that this would help me to build a solid financial future. I learned a lot from him. Even though I was hired to help him, he taught me some valuable lessons.

While working for the agency I learned that getting material things isn't the most important part of life. Many of our clients faced life without a roof over their heads. Some had problems with their feet, from living out in the rain, snow and bitter cold. But through all of their struggles, most continued to hold their heads high. Some of them were musicians and actors. They went to auditions and performed at venues. Most planned to find some kind of work and, eventually, housing. They had goals, hopes and dreams. One of them even showed me his business plan. He hoped to build his own company.

The job enabled me to give of my gifts, but also showed me the strength that all human beings have. If my clients could survive on so little, what could I do with the abundance I'd been given?

I decided that I could – and should – improve the lives of others and inspire them to find hope.

God continues to enable me to make a difference. He's taken away my darkness and helped me to see the potential we all have. What can you contribute? Can you help someone today? If you were kind and gave freely of your time and talent, would you be happier? If you develop an attitude of sharing you'll find that others will help you too.

The key to a happy life is to use your gifts and talents to help others. Look for ways to do so. Your outlook will improve when you help someone else. It may only be a small gift but it might mean a great deal to someone.

My babysitter asked me a question as I was writing this. She wondered if I could help her find film for her old camera. I stopped writing and found what she needed online. Then I bought it for her. She's done so much to help my family that she deserves all the kindness I can show her. This small gesture made her happier – and it made me happier too!

It would be great to live in a world in which everyone helps each other. There'd be no room for isolation or desperation. Your gift might be teaching, guiding, loving – or just listening. You can start to improve your life today by sharing what you have, one step at a time.

Blake LeVine

12: Choosing Faith over Darkness

One Friday morning I woke up in my usual way: I thanked God that I was alive and had been given the gift of another day. I was truly grateful, but I also had a problem: I only had a few dollars left in my bank account to get me and my family through the weekend.

My daughter was scheduled to participate in a preschool graduation celebration. The plan was for her and her three best friends to go out with my wife and the other mothers to have fun. I knew that if I told my wife that I was low on money she'd be upset. She sometimes gets upset over money matters because her parents often quarreled about their finances.

I decided not to argue. I had a few dollars that I'd saved during the week. I gave them to her for the celebration. I was concerned about getting through the weekend on what was in the account, but asked God for help and then let it go.

As the day went on, I spent time with my newborn son. We played in the kiddie pool and took a walk. When the mail arrived, I went to the mailbox to get it. How would God answer my prayer for help? In with the rest of the mail was a check for $400 – more than enough money to get us through the weekend! There was no need to worry or argue. I was thankful and winked at the sky.

If I'd told my wife that we were short on money – and fought with her about it – this check wouldn't have made a difference. We would have been angry with each other anyway. The choice I made was between faith and darkness. When you have faith in God and ask him to provide for your needs, things usually work out.

There are reasons why things happen the way they do. That weekend taught me that my wife and I had to do a better job of budgeting our money. We needed to work as a team to manage it in a responsible way. It isn't about being right or winning a fight, but learning to be responsible. When you have a family it's important to act like an adult. The responsible kind.

Claudia

Claudia is in her early thirties and has two young children. She's struggled with depression and addiction to painkillers. She was homeless for a time, but when we met her dad was letting her live in his home.

Claudia was going through a rough time. An electrical storm had knocked out the power in her father's house, so she had to move out and was living temporarily with her aunt. Her children were upset by the move, which added to her worries. We talked about how she needed to develop a positive outlook in spite of her current situation.

During the week that she lived with her aunt, Claudia examined her life and created a plan to accomplish her goals. She also took her two daughters swimming each day and focused her energy on her family. I asked her how she kept herself happy even though she'd had to leave her home.

Claudia told me that she decided not to let small problems upset her. She didn't let darkness into her life because doing so doesn't solve anything. She chose to make the best of things by living with her aunt and working with an electrician to get the power back at her father's house. Claudia said that she'd been through much worse: there had been times when she had no home, a horrible addiction and no money for food. Her current problems were small by comparison.

It's clear that she's a survivor. Although it was a hectic week for her, Claudia made time to participate in a coaching session with me. I was happy that she kept her appointment – it says a great deal about her character. Our session provided a healthy outlet for her to express her feelings. I believe that life will get easier for Claudia, and so does she. She's chosen to be optimistic about what's ahead.

Claudia told me that faith helps her to work through life's challenges. In the past she felt lost and alone when problems arose, and her addiction worsened. She used drugs to avoid facing up to challenges, and so they piled up and got worse. During her recovery she began to find hope in God.

She learned that prayer is a valuable tool in difficult times. She developed a relationship with God and believes that help is always available to her. She still has tough times, but now surrenders to God, asking for guidance and help. Claudia asked God to help her when the power went out. The answer she received was that it would all work out and that she should stay with her family. Knowing this, she was able to press on. She knew that she was not alone and could handle the situation.

Many people ask for proof that God exists, but faith means taking action when you don't have proof. Each of us is on a different journey. The lessons you learn might be different than those learned by others. This is why some people see God in everything while others do not believe at all.

Sometimes an overwhelming challenge motivates a person to seek God's help. A friend of mine, who is a Christian, wrote something interesting on his Facebook page. He wrote that he's a Christian because he's weak. He relies on God because he knows that he can't handle life without God's help. After experiencing a setback, only God can enable him to go on with his life

My friend's post tells me that his faith does not mean that he believes he is holier or better than anyone else. He suffered a setback and needed God to help him through it. There's no shame in needing help – certainly no shame in needing the help of something greater than yourself. If you have tried and failed in life, maybe you need something greater than your own abilities to set things right.

It's important for those who are struggling to recognize that the 12 steps are vital to recovery. During a group session at the rehab where I worked, I asked the participants about their faith and belief in God. Their responses varied. Some said that God had saved them and led them out of darkness. Others said there is no God – that it was all a lie. One person offered the opinion that we are all pieces of an exploding star.

I don't have all of the answers or the ability to prove one belief right and another wrong. But I know that faith has helped many through their difficulties. My brother's death did not destroy my love of life. Faith enabled me to process the loss and find comfort in my family.

I've seen God heal addicts, leading them away from their life-threatening habits. If faith helped them, why won't you give it a try? Sometimes people who've lived through tough times give up on God. They ask questions like why God would allow wars to be fought – wars in which innocent people are killed. I don't know the answer, but I believe that our pain can help us to learn and grow.

The loss of my brother has led me to celebrate each day, knowing that our time in this life is limited. His death taught me to value my life with my wife, children and the rest of my family. We don't know how much time we have left, so we shouldn't waste any of it.

I've also learned that it's necessary to care for others. When I work with an addict, I'm aware of how important the work is. If I can convince them to stop using, they won't die. That will be one family that won't have to suffer the loss that my parents and I live with.

I've become more confident as a result of Adam's death. I used to try to please everyone, but now I know that life is too precious – and short – to waste in this way. I have to do what's in my heart. It took almost three years for me to write my last book, and make it available to readers. But I knew that this book – the one you're reading – was needed NOW, so I allowed myself only a few months to get it to you.

Your decision – to accept faith or not – will be one of the biggest you ever make. Life has tested you, and you'll continue to run into obstacles. When you do, it can be easier to give in to darkness. The decision to end an addiction is harder to make. When you abuse drugs or sex, when you gamble, smoke or drink, you may not suffer the consequences until later. In the short term, it may seem like you're getting what you want or need.

But we know that these choices only create more problems. Look at the big picture: If you don't end an addiction it will end you. It's usually only after years of addiction that you can look back and see the damage it did, and continues to do. Addiction prevents you from accomplishing all that you can. You'll gain a lot of inner strength when you overcome it, and you'll find that your day-to-day life will be easier. You'll be proud of yourself for ending it. How would it feel if your experience helped someone who had a similar problem? You might give others the gift that enables them to rebuild their life.

The best friend I have is God. During rough times he's always there. When I come closer to him, he makes me feel confident, knowing that I'm not alone. He shows me how to find light during my darkest times. He never leaves me, even when it seems that everyone else has.

I've built a relationship with God that continues to inspire me. I've accepted that I have flaws and will always need to make changes. His love has taken my roughest experiences and turned them into tools to help others.

There's no greater joy than living your life to please God. I've learned to love others because God has helped me to love myself. I accept myself as I am, as he made me, and so I accept them as they are. I no longer try to be whoever I might think I'm supposed to be. God made all of us the way he wants us to be, and the experiences he's given us enable us to learn and grow.

13: Letting Go of the Old You

In the rehab where I worked, many clients shared a common problem: they had a hard time letting go of the life they'd been living. This included letting go of "friend" who could not be involved in their new life. They had a hard time letting go even when their past behavior – selling drugs, spending time in jail, hurting their loved ones – was toxic.

Some of them mourned the loss of their old life. They missed going to nightclubs, hanging out in bars and getting high. But it's only when you let go of your old life that you can begin to live a new one. I've known a lot of people who have moved on from the life they used to live to one that's healthier and more authentic. You can do it too.

Hugo

Hugo was a kind, honest man, who was addicted to opiates. He'd been through a lot in his 23 years. During treatment, Hugo admitted that much of what he'd done was wrong, including selling cocaine, physically abusing his mother and shooting a man who stole drugs from him.

Hugo was stuck. He had not completely faced his past, so he came to talk to me. I told him that the old Hugo was not the same person as the new one. The new Hugo doesn't hurt others, works on making his life better, and stays sober. Hugo agreed that he had made these changes. I also told him that he would have to let go of his old way of living – completely. This meant new friends, NA meetings and therapy. He would have to do all of it if he wanted to stay clean.

I sensed that Hugo missed his old life – that he mourned the loss of it as he would the loss of a friend. I knew that if he wanted to put his past behind him for good, he would have to bury his old self: the drug-dealing addict who did whatever he wanted.

Hugo needed to go slow and work hard. His days of fast living were over. He might not drive a Mercedes ever again, but he could live simply and well. He'd probably have to sell his jewelry to pay his drug debts. The women and friends who hung around him to get high would most likely disappear. But he'd end up in a better place.

It took a while, but Hugo finally accepted all of this. He knew that going back to his past would kill him. He was willing to move on. When he finished treatment, many who knew him didn't recognize him. His long hair and beard were gone. He walked instead of driving a fancy car. He couldn't be found at the strip club he used to frequent. The nights of getting high and going to Miami were over. Instead, he started taking care of his health and making better choices.

Hugo decided that he liked his new life. Now the people around him benefited from his kindness and friendship. He had nothing, in a material sense, to give anyone, so nobody used him. He went from having 100 "friends" to five real friends. His heart didn't race when he saw a police officer. He didn't worry that a drug addict might rob or kill him for his drugs.

I've found that small, simple gifts can be priceless. I took some time off from writing this book to take my son to a local park. He is eight months old today and loves being outside. When we got there, I put him in a small red swing. He smiled at me each time he swung back and forth. A beautiful yellow and black butterfly flew by us while we enjoyed the day. It was a blessing just to see him smile.

Later, we spent a few peaceful minutes in the shade of a big tree. It was amazing to watch him explore and discover the world. My son is just beginning life, so he has a clean slate. I hope he'll make good choices. I've also begun a new life. I've become closer to my family, and have found some wonderful friends who support the healthy choices I've made. I no longer drink, gamble, smoke or live with addictions. I no longer go to nightclubs or live a fast life. I'm proud to be a father, a coach and a productive member of our community.

This morning I went to a school to help the staff there learn how to better educate their students. I felt confident in who I am, and what I can do. A few years ago, I would have been nervous and struggled during the meeting. Accepting my true self has enabled me to be open to new experiences.

Nika

Nika was a beautiful young woman who lived a fast life. She worked as a stripper to pay for the fancy life she thought she deserved. She earned over $400,000 a year as a stripper and (sometimes) escort. She owned Balenciaga bags and Rolex watches. At first, she told herself that she liked her life. She had a lot of material things and met many rich men. She didn't think she would ever sleep with men for money, but eventually she did.

Nika began to experiment with drugs. Many of the strip club's customers used drugs when she was with them. Nika became addicted to crack. She stopped showing up for work on time and was fired when her appearance began to deteriorate.

Nika found out that she'd contracted a serious STD. The doctor told her that her overall health was failing. Her liver and kidneys had been badly damaged by the drugs she'd used and her other unhealthy habits.

That diagnosis woke her up. She stopped taking drugs, sought treatment and began to live differently. She could no longer afford to travel in limousines. It also became clear that she could no longer sell her body. Although it was sometimes scary for her to do so, Nika faced up to her challenges. She eventually began a career as a drug counselor. She returned to school and worked to pay her tuition.

Nika learned to love the simpler life she now lives. She likes to take hikes, read, watch educational documentaries and listen to music. Nika met a drug counselor who is also a recovering addict and they fell in love. She could talk to him about what she'd been through, telling him what she might be ashamed to tell others. He didn't care about her past – he had his own dark history. They went to NA meetings together and supported each other in recovery.

These days Nika travels widely, sharing her story with others. She is happy to have inspired others who were trapped in the sex industry to leave it and find a better life. She's taught high school students the importance of valuing their bodies. Nika loves being productive and making a positive impact in the world. She's let go of her past, and uses her experiences to help others who are stuck in the same traps.

Nika says that her life is happier than it's ever been. She no longer needs drugs to release pain, and knows that authentic love is the most valuable gift we can receive. When we honor our bodies and minds, we're able to feel authentic love, the kind that can't be bought, sold or traded.

Nika has seen what happens when you make bad choices. She hopes that others will not walk the hard road that she traveled. She is a blessing to others and is truly an inspiration.

Your old life is gone. Embrace the life you're living today. Things will be difficult when you first stop using drugs and alcohol. You may feel depressed about what you've lost – the partying, "friends" and all of the other things you once thought were "fun." But isn't it possible that there might be better things ahead for you? What would it be like to wake up every day feeling terrific? How about if you no longer lived in fear or regret? Would you like to be proud, confident and authentic? You aren't meant to live that old life. You'll have to make changes, but even small changes will help you to be happier.

You might feel lonely when you start to change your life. Sadly, when you change, you often need to change your friends too. Those who remain addicted cannot be your close friends. You'll relapse if you stay with people who are deep in addiction. Find a recovery group so you can spend time around people who are trying to accomplish exactly what you're working towards. You'll feel a sense of peace and calm when you do.

We – all of us – are influenced by the people we spend the most time with. Find yourself some hopeful, happy friends. You can walk into any NA or AA meeting in the world and feel a sense of community. In those rooms, they'll accept you no matter you've done. Spend your time with people who care, and who truly want to help you.

I've been blessed to be a guide for others. It's wonderful to watch them become what they're meant to be. I help them to understand why they decided to change, and to see the goals they're working towards. God helped me to change my life and to use what he taught me to help others.

In a way, it all makes sense: God puts us in a storm and helps us to work through it. Then he puts us back into the storm so that we use what we've learned to lead others out of it. Find people who can show you which way to go when you're caught in a storm. You don't need a lot of friends, only a few who can and will help you work through your challenges. One day you'll look back and be grateful that you found the support you needed to work through your problems.

A great teacher once told me that there are only a few outcomes for those who abuse drugs: jail, death or recovery. Don't go to jail for your addictions. Don't lose your life for them. Even if you've failed a hundred times, try recovery again. If you partner with someone who is dedicated to being your guide, you'll make progress.

The most important changes are often the most difficult. Will you let go of your past and take treatment seriously? If you do, there'll be no stopping you. You can achieve and maintain sobriety. All of the forces of darkness cannot stop you from living a clean life. If you let go of the old you, the new one will begin to emerge. I'm confident that the new you will be kind, smart, loving, compassionate and passionate. The light of your soul will begin to shine. We need your light.

14: Concrete Action

It seems obvious that we ought to set clear goals and work hard to achieve them. But we often become disoriented in the fog of day-to-day living and lose our focus. Going on Facebook, checking email, answering the phone – all of these and more distract us from what we've set out to accomplish.

Today I started my day in a wonderful way. After I woke, I spent an hour with my children at the park. Later, my mother came over to watch my daughter. When my son took a nap, I was free to begin work.

I started by putting together a checklist of what I wanted to accomplish. It included the three coaching sessions scheduled for today. It also included time to work on this book. I added some time to create content for our website. Other goals included mailing invoices, emailing clients, and preparing for the rest of the week.

When setting up a daily checklist I write the day and date on top, followed by what I need to accomplish on that day/date. As I complete each task, I check it off and move on to the next. My simple list of goals is almost always finished at the end of the day. I've learned to create a manageable list – one that is achievable. For example, with respect to my daily writing, it wouldn't be possible for me to write 15 chapters every day. At that rate I wouldn't have time to sleep! My current goal is one chapter a day. The chapters have averaged about 2,000 words each. At that rate, I'll finish the first draft in a week.

Since I've planned the book to contain 21 chapters, one per day will enable me to finish quickly. It takes me about two hours to write a chapter. When I work at this pace I'm able to balance the time I spend working on the book with time for friends and family. Trying to get it done faster would do more harm than good.

Dionne

Dionne was a 27 year old artist and poet. She said she felt "stuck" because she rarely completed her songs or drawings.

I asked her to describe how she worked. She told me that, when she felt like writing or drawing, she'd work for 8-10 hours in a manic burst. It felt sexy and exciting. But Dionne rarely finished what she started. She'd often be so tired the day after a creative burst that she stopped working altogether. She was frustrated because her work wasn't going anywhere. Her dream of earning a living as an artist seemed out of reach.

We had some great sessions, talking about her problem. I looked at samples of her work – her "beginnings." They were vibrant and intelligent: she's an amazing artist. I told her that art is, for some, a career and business. If she wanted to be one of those artists, she'd have to change her work habits and she'd have to create a plan.

We put together a schedule to bring some order to her creative process. Dionne decided to work on her art for three hours per day, three days a week. She'd keep working on projects until they were finished. She wouldn't allow herself to begin anything new until whatever she'd started was finished. In addition, she put together a plan to market her work. It included locating galleries, and sites where she could sell her work online. Dionne said that when she did these things her creative work began to feel like a real job. She started each day with a list of tasks to complete. She did them one at a time and, by the end of each day, finished most of them. Dionne completed several pieces of art, which gave her a sense of pride and accomplishment. Her work was accepted by three galleries, one of which was the site of her first show.

Dionne prepared properly and was ready to earn a living as an artist. She understood how much she'd helped herself by making concrete plans. She realized that successful artists must know what they're doing, in a practical way. They must master both the creative *and* business sides of the process. Dionne no longer gets so burnt out that she must stop working. She knows that by taking time and working steadily towards clear goals, she'll produce the best work that she can.

When you have a clear set of goals you're more likely to accomplish them. This is true of whatever you want to do. If you need to go to 60 recovery meetings in 60 days, make a list that shows what you need to do and when. When you go to a meeting, check it off the list. At a glance, you'll be able to tell how many meetings you've attended and how close you are to achieving your goal.

You can use the same approach to solve money problems. You might not know the exact amount necessary to pay off your debts, but if you take a few steps each day you'll find that, eventually, each bill will be repaid. These steps can include finding a job, building a business or lowering your expenses. Don't let fear of what you need to do overwhelm you. Break it down to simple steps, work on them every day, and you'll make progress. There's almost nothing you can't accomplish if you take a few steps towards it each day.

Matt

Matt was a talented teacher who was battling alcoholism and depression. He knew that he couldn't teach effectively when he was depressed or hung-over. Since he felt that education was his calling, he was willing to do whatever was necessary to be the best teacher he could be.

Matt began to live according to a schedule of therapy, medication and recovery meetings. After several months, he decided to build a freelance tutoring business. He knew that it would be easier for him to tutor 5 or 6 children a week, than to deal with classrooms full of students day after day. Matt determined that he could earn close to $800 per week by tutoring for about 25 hours. This would enable him to attend AA meetings and therapy, with time left over for hiking. Previously, when Matt would work at a school, the school administration would handle everything related to finances. When he started tutoring, this was no longer the case.

Matt set a goal to deliver his resume to two tutoring companies each day. In the first two weeks he visited over 15 of them. He had five interviews, which resulted in three job offers. Matt created an online calendar to track his tutoring sessions. He also created a chart that showed the payments that were due to him from each of the tutoring companies.

Matt saw the systems he put in place make his life easier. They even helped him to be a better teacher. He created folders on his computer in which he kept all of his notes and student assignments. He'd check the folders five minutes before each tutoring session to remind himself of what the student worked on the last time they met. He knew which tests and essays were due at each student's school.

The families who work with Matt love his professional approach. He hopes to eventually own his own tutoring company, and is laying the groundwork for that business. He knows that by taking these steps he'll be ready when the opportunity arises.

I used to feel that setting goals limited my freedom. My style was to handle whatever happened when it happened. When I became a father I knew this wouldn't work. I had to know ahead of time when my children had appointments, when to pick them up, and be aware of any changes in plan. My wife and I had to let each other know what was going on, and when.

One weekend my wife was going away to take a course. I needed to know when she'd leave, and when she'd be back – the days, dates and times. Together we prepared a schedule so I'd be ready to care for the children, business and household while she was away. I coordinated with my parents and my father-in-law to make plans for Father's Day. I knew what food I needed to buy, who'd be coming and when they'd arrive. Because I planned ahead, the day was enjoyable. I didn't have to figure it all out on the spot.

Planning is helpful, but things don't always go according to plan. I might have 10 goals set for today but then something changes. If my power went out during yesterday's rainstorm I wouldn't be able to finish everything I wanted to accomplish. And when, for example, your child is sick, that overrules everything else.

The key is to be flexible: deal with what comes, then get back on track as quickly as possible.

If the power went out yesterday, I'd take whatever I didn't finish on yesterday's list and move it to today's. "A day late" is still "finished." I've seen many clients get thrown off their schedules for months when something unexpected arises.

After my brother died I had to pick up where I left off. The week I spent with family was focused on grieving and being with my loved ones. I didn't do any work. The following week I went back to my job at the rehab and worked with my private clients. It helped to have a routine and to be productive. If I'd sat at home doing nothing I would have become more depressed. I know my brother was happy that I went to work and helped others who struggle with addiction. Over the next few weeks, my clients and I enjoyed some wonderful moments. It was healing to know that I was doing something positive during a sad time in my life.

You may find that when you come up against problems, even your best plans must change. All of us sometimes encounter situations that stop us cold. You have to deal with them, but don't give up on what you wanted to accomplish no matter what happens. It's never too late to pick up where you left off.

I met a friend who encouraged me to start writing again. At the time, I was so busy that I couldn't even consider starting a new book. But her encouragement led me to begin writing this – the book you're reading – and I'm glad that it did. It's been a release for my energies and, hopefully, I've shared some valuable lessons with you. I've been reminded how much fun it is to finish a book. Seeing it in print gave me a lot of satisfaction. I'm excited that others will read it and pray that it will inspire you to find happiness.

Writing this book has helped me deal with something I didn't see coming. The last time I saw my brother I hoped that he'd move in with me, that we'd spend our days together. I never thought that less than a year later he'd be dead. We never know what will happen to us, but I believe we can press on, no matter what. You can take your biggest problem and use it to turn your life around. Facing big challenges is a way to learn and grow.

15: Listen To Your Heart

Do you listen to your inner voice? It's a good idea to do so when you need to make a difficult decision. I used to do what I wanted, even when my heart told me to do something else. Now I understand that my inner voice is almost always correct.

Each species has certain abilities that enable it to survive. Some have a strong sense of smell or hearing that helps them to be aware of danger. Most creatures rely on their special skills and don't second-guess them. If you listen to your inner voice you'll make better decisions.

Inga

Inga is a thirty year old woman who was addicted to alcohol, marijuana and cigarettes. She used these addictions to block out what her inner voice told her. She was in a relationship with an alcoholic who was angry and sometimes violent. He'd hit her and then try to make up with her, buying flowers and taking her to dinner. Inga lived in a constant state of fear. She didn't love her boyfriend but reasoned that he was the best she could do. Inga didn't earn much as a haircutter and knew it would be hard to survive without his financial help. The breaking point arrived in the form of a big argument. Inga's boyfriend broke her nose. As the blood rushed out, she knew that the relationship was over.

Inga worked on becoming strong and valuing herself. She came to believe that she's beautiful and kind, and deserves to be with a healthy man. Inga stopped using substances and became a frequent attendee at AA meetings. She found a sponsor and met others who had survived abusive relationships.

Inga learned to trust her inner voice. She relied on it when she began dating. If she was uncomfortable with a man she wouldn't see him again. It took a long time, but she eventually made some big changes in her life. She got her own apartment, made some new friends and developed a strong sense of her self-worth.

Inga met a strong, sensitive man named Jorge. He respected women and treated Inga with kindness. Jorge is also in recovery. Together they've built a warm, supportive relationship. She feels comfortable with him; he encourages her. They go on hikes, travel and go to movies. Previously, Inga worried that her boyfriend might be angry or violent with her. She was always on edge, because she wasn't sure what would happen. But her relationship with Jorge is one of mutual respect and love. They help each other and work through problems together.

Pratt

Pratt is an 18 year old man who always wanted to be in control. He grew up in a mansion in Brentwood, California. His dad was a famous director who's always busy. His mom was self-absorbed and left Pratt with a nanny for most of his early life. At his posh private school, Pratt made friends who also came from rich families and had lots of money. When he was 12, one of Pratt's friends introduced him to drinking.

Pratt started drinking vodka, beer and whiskey. He thought that it was cool and it helped him to bury his feelings. Pratt thought that his family only cared about their careers and social lives – not him. Drinking helped him to numb his depression.

Pratt stopped going to school and was eventually expelled. His parents finally expressed concern, but only because he'd embarrassed them. They sent him to a boarding school for troubled youth in Massachusetts. This turned out to be a horrible decision. The students snuck in drugs and Pratt became addicted to heroin. The other students sometimes beat him up.

Even though he came from a wealthy background, he was morally bankrupt. His anger and addictions created a hailstorm of pain. Pratt overdosed and woke up to some serious legal difficulties. He'd hit a dog while driving intoxicated. Pratt was arrested for driving under the influence and was remanded to treatment.

Pratt admitted that he never listened to his inner voice. Years earlier he felt that he needed to stop his addiction. He knew that he should talk to his parents and tell them how angry he was because he felt they had abandoned him. He knew that much of his self-destructive behavior was due to not following his heart.

Pratt and I worked together to help him listen to his inner voice. He began to think about where his path in life might lead, and about who he truly was. He no longer felt the need to live in Brentwood and be around people who are focused on fame and money. He decided to find a career that would support him financially and enable him to do something productive with his life.

Pratt returned to school and studied water conservation. He got a job in Georgia at a nature preserve. Today Pratt lives a simple and abundant life. He educates people about the importance of water. He also made new friends who love and accept him.

Together they go on hikes, eat dinner and create a sense of community.

Pratt made peace with his parents. His dad had a breakdown and now lives a simpler life. He and Pratt have grown their relationship – they see each other three times a year. Pratt accepted his inner calling to live in a simple way. He's not afraid of having little money. For him, money is only useful for providing basic necessities. He followed his heart and is living his own truth.

We often know which path we should follow, but knowing doesn't always make it easier to take the right steps. My son Ryan is 8 months old. When we moved from Los Angeles to Florida we didn't have health insurance. It was a mistake, but we didn't take him to the doctor for his six-month checkup. I reasoned that he probably didn't need it, but if he did, maybe I didn't want to know why. I didn't want to consider the possibility that he might have a serious problem.

Ryan became constipated. He struggled to go to the bathroom – it caused him a lot of discomfort. My parents pressured me to take him to the doctor. They even offered to pay, which left me no way to avoid it.

We arrived early for the appointment. I filled out several pages of paperwork. When we went into the exam room we were met by a nursing assistant, then the doctor came in. While she examined him, Ryan smiled and laughed. She told us that he was within the healthy weight and height ranges, and was on-track in terms of his developmental goals. She gave Ryan four vaccinations – he only cried a little bit. I left the office happy and relieved. The doctor said his constipation was likely due to his diet. She recommended a different formula and more solid food.

My inner voice told me not to be afraid to take him to the doctor. I saw that I was being a poor father by not seeking help. I always advised my clients to seek help but was scared to bring my child to the doctor. My inner voice told me that it's always better to face a situation than to ignore it.

How many of us avoid doing what we need to do? We allow fear to prevent us from doing what's necessary. I'm continuing to learn that this doesn't have to be the case. Fear is based on perception. Sometimes what scares us most turns out to be nothing to be afraid of. Many people refuse treatment for addictions or mental health problems because they worry about what they'll have to deal with.

It was hard for me to admit that I was delusional and hallucinating when I was a teenager. I worried that others would find out and lock me up in a mental hospital. My fears became real when I didn't deal with the situation properly.

When I listened to my inner voice and accepted that I needed treatment my life improved. I admitted that I was sick and that it was important for me to get the medications and therapy that I needed. Once I accepted that I needed help, I began to recover. I found the right medications and a terrific therapist. I no longer suffer from these problems.

My inner voice tells me that I wouldn't be the healthy father and husband I am if I hadn't sought help. It's scary to admit that you have a serious health problem, but the good news is that when you seek help, you can overcome it. Hiding your addiction will not make it go away. Even while hidden, the problem continues to grow. I believe we can overcome almost any difficulty if we take the small, slow steps necessary to change our lives.

Maybe you feel as if there's a mountain in your way. Maybe it's addiction, mental illness, financial problems, relationship issues or isolation. Your inner voice tells you to get help because you won't be able to climb over it on your own. I've seen people end their lives rather than seek help.

I've worked with clients who've killed people while high, lost their families and faced other problems. One of them spent 20 years in jail for killing a friend while he was on drugs. He found God in jail, and made it through his term. When he got out, he was ready to rebuild his life. He found a job, an apartment, friends and even a wife. Today he lives a full life even though he did something horrible. He served his time in jail, asked God for forgiveness and decided to press on. He sponsors other addicts and shares his story with them. If he could overcome all of that, can't you overcome your problem? Take the first step: seek help.

Your inner voice is always there to help you. Listen to it. It will likely tell you who you're meant to be. I've seen people evolve and grow. They find happiness in living a full life when they discover who they really are. If you take this journey you'll eventually arrive at a place of hope, encouragement, peace, friendship and love.

16: Pass the Test

During my years of schooling I've taken a lot of tests. I usually did well because I stayed calm. Many bright students do poorly, because they get so nervous that they lose their grip on what they know. Being able to center yourself will help you pass the tests you face.

I recently spent my first Fathers' Day with my new son. During the week that led up to it I had to pass several tests. One of them was to remain calm as my wife, who was depressed, told me how unhappy she was in Florida. We have a wonderful home there, our children have many friends, we've met several nice couples and my career has blossomed.

I spoke quietly with her about all of this. She told me that she misses her mother, who passed away several years ago. Living in Florida, where her mom lived and died, has been hard for her. During our discussion I had a disagreement with her, but quickly told her I was sorry. We agreed that happiness should not be defined by where you live and that there are many positive aspects to our current life. We both know that, even if we moved, she'd still have to deal with her depression.

She made an appointment to speak with a doctor. A change in medication may help her. Previously, when she took antidepressants, her quality of life was much better. I was tested by her negativity, but gave her time to search her soul and realize that she needs help. I didn't get angry just because we'd hit some turbulence. That's how to pass a test.

I've been helping my wife watch our children. She'd been anxious about a big test she had to take as part of her physician assistant training. We didn't have the $1,000 fee for the study course, hotel and other expenses of the trip to the test site. She told me about this just a few weeks before she needed to leave.

Jennifer had to complete the class and earn her Florida license in order to keep her job. We decided that she could stay for free at my uncle's home in Orlando (where the class would be held). I agreed to babysit both children for the three days she'd be away. This would be the first time I'd watch the new baby alone for this length of time.

It turned out that my wife's dad offered to pay for the class and the hotel. They decided to make a father-and-daughter weekend out of it, and he drove her to the class. That's how they celebrated Father's Day.

I found out later that, as part of their plans, I would watch my father-in-law's golden retriever. He's a beautiful dog, but wild. This meant that I'd be supervising two dogs, a cat, fish, my eight-month-old son and five-year-old daughter. I'd have to walk the dogs, clean the house, feed everyone, get up to take care of the baby in the middle of the night, etc., etc.

I made the best of the arrangement and passed my test. My son woke me up four times during the night. When we went to breakfast the next morning he had an attack of diarrhea at the International House of Pancakes. But I passed my test.

The following morning he woke me at 5:30. I went downstairs and saw that I'd have to clean up after the dog. Some of the padding that we'd put on the floor so that the baby could practice crawling was drenched in urine and had to be thrown away. I scrubbed the floor. Afterwards, my feet and hands smelled of urine. The day had just begun but I passed my test by not becoming angry or upset.

It was a long weekend. I did my best to stay calm and enjoy the days. Once I had to drive someone to the train station. I brought the two kids with me. While I put them in the car it was raining so hard that I got drenched. I accidentally dropped my keys somewhere in the backseat. The rain dripped off me as I searched for them.

I told the person who I was taking to the train station that I was blessed to have kids. Many people try for years to have children but are not successful. I was grateful to be able to watch them on Father's Day weekend. I smiled through each test as it was presented to me. As I passed each of them, they became less difficult. That evening my dad watched my daughter for four hours and my son fell asleep, so I took a shower and was able to write for a while. When you pass your tests, positive results follow.

Some people resort to drinking or drugs when they're tested, but more problems arise when they do so. I couldn't have passed my tests if I was drunk or high. I would have passed out or become violent. I took these tests with a large dose of faith. I asked God for help each time difficulties arose and gave thanks when I handled things successfully. I know that I'm blessed, even during hard times. Each experience is an opportunity to learn. God has a plan for all of us and I have learned to trust him.

Wilma

Wilma was a 27-year-old who worked with her parents. Their company sold motors for electric scooters. It took her grandfather and dad many years to build the business. Wilma started in sales and slowly worked her way up through the company. She was driven and dedicated to making her family's company a success.

Wilma's brother was an alcoholic, but her family overlooked his problem. When he was appointed CEO of the company, she was hurt, but didn't tell anyone how she felt. He seemed to work hard, but often missed deadlines. Wilma's brother eventually caused the business to lose its two biggest clients. The company edged close to bankruptcy.

Wilma begged her dad to let her take over – to give her a chance to turn the company around. She felt that she'd proven that she was up to the challenge. Her dad said no, but she persisted. She worked hard and landed two new clients. The business began to grow again. It took five more years but her brother was eventually pushed out of the company. Wilma became the first female CEO in her family's business.

Wilma is now a successful executive, leading her family's company into the future. Under her leadership, the business has grown from $8 million in sales to over $100 million. Wilma never gave up and passed her test. These days she receives the respect and appreciation she deserves. It took years of patience, but she says it was worth the wait.

Clint

Clint was a heroin addict who wanted to stop using, but something always seemed to get in the way of his recovery. He'd quit for a day, then something horrible would happen. He'd relapse and go back to using. He lost his job, his wife left him, he was arrested, his home was broken into, and he was robbed at gunpoint. Clint began to feel that heroin was his only choice. He was failing his test because his addiction made it so hard for him to pass.

If it was easy to stop using drugs, there wouldn't be so many addicts. It often gets harder just when you try to stop.

Clint admitted that he was dying – that he was killing himself. He knew that he would, unless he was able to change. We worked on his problems together, and he stopped using. When obstacles arose he remained calm and called me to talk about them. We'd discuss his feelings, and he was able to avoid relapsing.

Clint had stopped using for four days when his mother was diagnosed with a brain tumor. She was the one person in his life who helped and encouraged him. He was angry and told me that he wanted to get high. I said that if he did it would not only hurt him, it would hurt his mom. I asked him to pray for help. He did. Clint asked God to help his mom, and to keep him away from heroin. He said this was the hardest test he'd ever taken.

Clint remained off drugs and helped his mom deal with her diagnosis. Eventually, she made a full recovery. These days Clint and his mom enjoy each other. She's happy that he's off heroin. Her biggest fear was losing him to an overdose. His biggest fear was that the tumor would kill her. They both overcame their fears and helped each other make it through hard times.

Clint knows that he passed his final exam. He's finally free from addiction. I think it was killing his mom too, and that her fears for him were part of the reason why she became sick. When Clint and his mother chose faith in God they saw their lives turn around. It's beautiful when good people pass big tests. The right decision can provide the hope and healing you want – and need.

17: A New Outcome

You might worry that past choices have led you to take a dangerous path through life. When you abuse drugs or alcohol, it puts every aspect of your life at risk. But you can get a different outcome if you're willing to change your behavior. One of the keys to healing is believing that you can get different results. Better results. You might not understand how that can happen, but many of your past problems were brought on by addiction. Remove addiction from the picture and things can get better fast. It often starts with changing your expectations.

Paulina

Paulina was a former Marine who lived life to the fullest. She was confident, physically fit and motivated. But when her father died from a rare blood disorder, she became angry that God would do such a thing to her and fell into depression. Paulina couldn't find any happiness in the life she used to love. She began drinking wine. What started with a glass or two developed into a major addiction. It wasn't long before she'd shake all over when she needed a drink. She began to drink just to get through the day.

One of Paulina's cousins, frightened by her steady decline, came to talk to her. He told Pauline how she had been someone he looked up to. She'd been strong and energetic – someone who was never afraid. He told her that now it looked to him as if her love of life was gone.

Paulina was shocked and upset by what her cousin told her. She realized that her problem was a big one and, unless she did something about it, it would get worse. She decided to see a psychiatrist and also began to meet with me for therapy.

Together, we explored her feelings. Paulina admitted that she was angry with God, and with her dad. Why did God let her get so close to her dad, then take him away from her before she told him how important he was to her?

I told Paulina that her anger was ruining her life. She'd have to choose: move on, or die. Paulina began a long journey of self-discovery and healing. The medications she took for depression helped remove the gloom and darkness from her eyes. It took a while, but Paulina began to feel happier.

Once she started to make progress I helped Paulina to expect a new outcome. A better outcome. Years of drinking had left her believing that things would always fall apart for her. I helped her to set goals and expect happiness – to feel optimistic about her plans. Paulina decided that she wanted to be a nursing assistant. She also wanted to begin dating, and to join the National Guard. This last goal would enable her to work in the structured environment in which she'd thrived, but in a more relaxed way.

Paulina expected her plans to succeed and, eventually, they did. She met a handsome man who loves her very much. She no longer drinks, and deals with stress holistically (exercise, deep breathing, long hikes, etc.). She started to exercise so that she'd be strong enough to handle her work with the Guard.

It's been a long, hard road for Paulina, but she's stronger and wiser because she made good decisions. She accepted the loss of her dad. She realized that being happy is what he'd want her to do. He would be proud that she sought help and eventually found her passion. Paulina says she speaks to his spirit, and that she'll continue to honor him by making good choices.

You'll enjoy many benefits when you live a healthier life. I recently took a two-hour hike in a local nature preserve. It helped me to connect with my surroundings and to appreciate the beauty that God has created.

My simple decision – to take this hike – provided other benefits that might not be obvious. The exercise strengthened my body. The opportunity to relax enabled me to release stress. I was able to center myself and let go of frustration and fear.

I always expect wonderful outcomes in my life. This doesn't mean that I believe that every situation will go my way. I know that sometimes what I want is not what's best for me. I hope for things to go as I would like, but have learned to adjust when my plans are not met.

I once listened to someone talk about a lesson he'd learned. He said that a man told him how easy it must be for him (the speaker) to be happy. He's wealthy, successful and helps others. The speaker told his audience that his life hadn't always been this way. It became a joy only after he learned to focus on what was good about it. Now, even when he faces difficult challenges, he doesn't feel pessimistic.

I know what he meant. I just lived through the loss of my only brother, my grandmother, and a stroke suffered by my other grandmother – all in a short period of time. It wasn't easy, but I decided to see what I could learn from the experience. Instead of denying my feelings and escaping into drug or alcohol abuse, I made a different choice. I asked God for his love and support, and have found outlets for me that include writing, rapping, hiking and playing tennis. I feel pure happiness when I spend time with my children. I've reconnected with my parents and have supported them during this tough time. I haven't allowed pain to harden my heart or make my light grow dim. I believe that there are even more great experiences ahead for me.

Vic

Vic was recovering from opiate addiction. He told me that recovery was the hardest and most complicated battle he'd ever fought. Vic said that NA helped him to accept his life, and that he found community and encouragement at the meetings. He also found a great sponsor who was always available to help him.

Vic believed that he wouldn't have survived without the support of his local group. He became a leader and helped others with their recovery. The positive changes he experienced began to benefit others who were still fighting addiction. They gave him the courage to keep moving forward.

When I make positive choices I help myself, but also hope that my experiences will help others. I'm blessed to be able to use my experiences to educate. I could have rotted away in depression and addiction but I expected something different. Something better. I asked God to heal me and decided that I'd never give up on my life. I'm often tested, and do my best to make good choices. Still, I sometimes make bad decisions.

I know that I'm not perfect. That's o.k., as long as I learn from my mistakes. I'm a very different person from the one I used to be. I try hard to do right and help others. If you know someone who never makes mistakes please, let me know how I can get in touch with him or her. I'd love to meet and learn from such a person.

People with good hearts always try to do the best they can. Being an addict doesn't make you a bad person. Many people turn to drugs and alcohol to deal with stress. It has been harder for me to avoid drugs and alcohol than it would have been to use them.

I see liquor every day – in grocery stores, restaurants and private homes. I'm often around people who are drinking. My dad used to drink each night and claimed it was just to have "fun." When I was younger I drank socially. It was fun to go out and party. It's been harder to make friends since I stopped drinking, but I feel healthier and more confident.

At the same time, I've continued to face the challenges that many of my clients face. When my brother died it would have been easy to drink to numb my pain. During other stressful times it would have been easy to drink, just to calm down. These are the reasons why so many people struggle with sobriety. The good news is that when you make better choices, you'll get a better outcome: a life of God, hope, happiness, healing and health. You'll hold onto your gifts when you give up drinking, and maybe find some that you never knew you had.

Finding support is vital to recovery. NA and AA have done an amazing job, helping millions of people to be reborn. They ask for no money and seek no publicity. Quietly, they man the front lines in communities around the world.

There are also amazing organizations helping those who suffer from mental illness. *The National Alliance on Mental Illness* and *The Depression and Bipolar Support Alliance* have hundreds of local support groups. They offer their assistance free to anyone impacted by mental health problems.

I would not have made it through my battle with mental illness without support groups. Since my recovery, they've welcomed me to share my books and lessons with their clients. I'm grateful to the local leaders who devote their time and abilities to these groups. They are the heroes you never hear about. I encourage you to find a group and participate.

When you do your part AND work with others you develop your mind and body, and will likely be rewarded with a good outcome. It's never too late to turn your life towards that outcome. It doesn't matter where you are: please seek help. You don't need to fight this battle alone – and you shouldn't. You're more likely to find and use the resources you need with the help of others. If you want to learn more about the organizations I've mentioned, visit the following websites:

- Narcotics Anonymous: www.na.org
- Alcoholics Anonymous: www.aa.org
- Depression and Bipolar Support Alliance: www.dbsaalliance.org
- The National Alliance on Mental Illness: www.nami.org

18: Depression and Addiction

The past several years have been difficult ones for a lot of people. Due to the economic downturn, many have lost jobs, homes and more. Families and individuals suffered – some of them suffered from depression. And many of those who did made their problems worse by making bad choices. Sadly, some decided to combat depression with alcohol, marijuana, cocaine, ecstasy, opiates and other substances.

My history has given me some insights into the problem. I went through several rough years when I struggled financially while dealing with emotional problems. I lost my brother, grandmother and others who were close to me. I used to think that having a drink to calm my nerves was a helpful thing to do, but I realized that it didn't help at all. Instead, I chose faith.

My journey began when I started listening to motivational talks, including some by Joel Osteen and Wayne Dyer. They sustained my soul. I was lonely, and these speakers became the inspirational friends I desperately needed.

My relationship with God grew stronger. Previously, I'd ask for his help only when serious problems arose. I learned that I need God every day. I prayed often, and slowly became someone who surrounds himself with positivity, inspiration and faith. Now I listen to religious radio stations in the car and watch motivational videos on YouTube every day.

When my brother died I chose not to sink into addiction and instead relied on inspiration. I've actually become a happier person since he passed away. I miss him, but have accepted the reality of death and no longer fear it. We'll all be gone some day; it's vital to celebrate life while we have it. One of the best ways to do that is to honor God.

I've developed a winning attitude. Most successful people know the importance of staying positive and motivated. God's encouragement will enable you to persist even when it seems like you can't. You'll never wake up feeling sick after a night of prayer.

My beliefs were confirmed during a visit to a psychic. He told me that my brother had chosen to numb his pain with drugs and alcohol, but I should rely on faith instead. He said that if I did so, I'd inspire others by my example.

When you're battling hard times, please choose faith. It's the one thing you can lean on and know that it won't let you fall. It's not a temporary fix, but a lifetime friendship with God.

Lucy

Lucy lost her job in the music industry. She missed working for the record label, which made her feel successful. Her boyfriend lost his job too, so money was short. They left Los Angeles and moved to New Jersey, close to family. Lucy felt like a loser. She no longer spent her days with famous musicians, partying and living a glamourous life. She started drinking wine and smoking marijuana, and her relationship with her boyfriend became tense.

While discussing their problems, Lucy's boyfriend encouraged her to ask God for help. He told her that she had to stop using drugs and alcohol, and see a psychiatrist. Lucy began a medication regimen and attended services at a local temple. It took some time, but her life got better. She found that with hope and faith she could deal with her problems.

Lucy and her boyfriend started an online company to help people with depression. It became popular and received funding from large investors. She became a business leader who often spoke to groups about these topics. Eventually she sold the company for over $500 million.

Today Lucy is a happy, dynamic – and blessed – woman. She vacations all over the world and is happy that she fought the good fight of faith. Lucy knows that her experiences led her to help others who face the same problems.

At one time or another we'll all face tough situations. In the past, you may have chosen to numb your feelings with drugs and alcohol, but the best recipe for dealing with depression is a simple one. Mix faith, inspiration, hope, treatment, friendships, family and love. When you combine these ingredients you're likely to end up with a great outcome. One day look you'll look back and be grateful that you made the more difficult choice.

When I collected autographs I thought that famous people had it all. I believed that they could do whatever they wanted to do, whenever they wanted to do it. They must be happy all of the time. I met many stars, but began to notice that some were dead broke even though they had, at one time, earned lots of money. Others were miserable and selfish, blinded by their big egos.

There are plenty of happy celebrities, but fame and wealth are not necessarily a ticket to happiness. If joy is what you want, find it in being motivated, having a good purpose, true friends, family, and a relationship with God. Don't bother looking for it in drugs or alcohol. You won't find it there.

You CAN change. You may be depressed, focusing on what's gone wrong. It's up to you to deal with those feelings. If you're willing to retrain your brain you can believe that life is great.

Our brains believe what they're taught. A beautiful woman can look in a mirror and see someone who's fat or ugly. Practice telling yourself something simple – you're a success, you're overcoming your addiction, you are happy, life is wonderful, God loves you. Say it to yourself several times a day. Before long, your brain will believe it. Trust me – it works.

Life doesn't always have to be hard. One way to make it easier is to get the support you need. My coaching practice offers a program for those who suffer from depression, addiction and other mental health challenges. Visit **BipolarOnline.com** to learn how we can help you. We work directly with all of our clients and every one of them has made progress.

I've never gone without food or been homeless. I've enjoyed financial success while learning the importance of sharing. I'm grateful for all I've been given, and I'm willing to help in bigger ways. I know how important it is to take my own advice. My skills have become so ingrained in my personality that being happy is easy!

As you read this you might feel that you have a lot of work to do. Take small steps. You don't have to be perfect: never angry, sad or frustrated. All of us face hardship – the key is to not let it prevent you from working towards your goals.

Many people have successfully dealt with problems they didn't think they could solve. They find ways to remain hopeful while they keep working. They have a relationship with God that's strong enough to survive hard times. God doesn't guarantee that things will be perfect, but with faith you'll make it through the storm. What you learn along the way may someday help someone else.

19: Lemons into Lemonade

When I was a boy my mother always turned lemons into lemonade. It's her favorite expression and she lives by it. My mom has survived some tough times, including growing up with a mother who was often toxic and negative. While raising me, there were times when she was broke. She lost me for a while when my dad kidnapped me. She had a rough marriage and divorce. She stood by me during my many psychiatric hospital stays and throughout my rebellious years.

My mom lost her son to a heroin overdose. She lost her mom in the same year. During this time she also had to deal with moving and financial problems. If she became angry or hostile I'd have to admit that she'd earned the right to feel that way. But she continues to stay positive and enjoy life.

These days she helps us to take care of her grandchildren, plays tennis, spends time with friends and is building a new therapy practice (she's a therapist too). She doesn't allow my brother's death and the other hardships she's suffered to hold her back. She's an eternal optimist who has passed this gift on to me.

One of the reasons why I've been successful as a therapist – and as a human being – is because I find the bright side in every situation. All of us are free to decide how we'll handle what we experience. I always choose to make the best of it.

The book (and film) *Silver Linings Playbook* presents characters who find ways to help each other when their lives are touched by bipolar disorder. One of the actresses in the film is named Jennifer Lawrence. That's an interesting coincidence for me because my wife is Jennifer and my dad's name is Lawrence! He wanted to name me Lawrence Jr. but my mom refused because in Judaism father and son don't share the same first name.

Look for the silver lining. Always.

Can you see the bright parts of your life? Are you willing to focus on the good and let go of past pain? There's good in your life today. You're a survivor. You've struggled, but here you are, reading this and (I hope) learning from it. You're alive now – you've been given the gift of being in this moment. Just by thinking about changing your life you've proven that you want to do it. You're unique, beautiful and valuable, and you have gifts to share with the world. God made you just as he wanted you to be. He believes in you and will help you to make better choices.

Here's something that I want to share with you. When I was younger I often made bad decisions. I did what I wanted – not what God wants. And so I had problems and lived with anxiety and fear. As I came closer to God my life got better. I still have problems – the difference is that now I see and respond to them differently.

I'm selling a property that I own in New York City. We found a buyer and prepared the contract. Then I got a call from my real estate agent who told me that the buyer was, maybe, not going to move forward on the deal.

I had plans for the money from the sale – I was depending on it being completed – but I told the realtor it would all work out. We laughed about how she acts as a therapist to many buyers and sellers who tell her about their problems. I told her that I was sure we'd find the right buyer. I was sure that by the time this book was released the apartment would be sold. My attitude turned around what many would call "bad news."

How we handle situations is up to us. In this instance, I made an executive decision. I could have called my parents, friends or wife (or all of them) and whined. If I had, I would have made them feel bad – just because I was disappointed. Who knows, they might have been having a great day until I called, but not after I got done with them. I don't want to bring others down with by whining and complaining. I'd rather build people up.

Of course you need outlets for your problems. I speak to my therapist about difficult situations I'm dealing with. I trust him and know that he'll help me work through them. The difference is that therapists are trained to listen and respond honestly. It's harder – sometimes impossible – for family and friends to do this impartially.

When I decided that I wanted to move from New York to Los Angeles, I knew that my mom would be upset about it. I asked a therapist to help me decide what was best – stay or go. I struggled to find the most painless way to break the news to my mother, and to work through it with her.

My mom was sad when I told her I'd decided to leave, but once again she made lemons out of lemonade. She kept our bond strong by talking with me on the phone every day. We remained close and, eventually, both of us moved to Florida. Now I see her often and we spend holidays together as one big family.

You should work with a guide who is honest and cares about you, and is also impartial. My team and I are here to help you. You can reach us anytime at **(213) 304-9555**. We'll show you how to find the bright side of whatever you're facing. Our goal is to teach you the amazing lesson my mom instilled in me: how to take lemons and make lemonade.

Blake LeVine

20: Your New Start

It's been almost 20 years since I was a psychiatric patient, lying awake at night, thinking about how good it would be to be free. I made a new start on life when I found the right medications and therapy.

Today I have a beautiful wife and two amazing children. I've written several books which have been published – doing so had been one of my dreams. I've started a business, which is thriving. I've made films that have been optioned by a major Hollywood producer. I've spoken in front of large audiences around the world, sharing my message of hope. Most importantly, I spend my days happy and fulfilled. I've found a life of purpose and service to God.

I'm sharing this – bragging about it – to make a point. When I was depressed, all of the blessings I now enjoy seemed far away. Unreachable. Back then, I might have been called 'unstable' for believing that one day I'd be blessed in these ways. But I've learned to hold onto my dreams, no matter what others might think.

I believe in slow, steady progress. Almost anything is possible if you take small steps, slowly. I've taken those steps, and they've taken me a long way. You can take them too.

Don't give up on yourself. The goals that you once had – that were once important to you – can be yours again. It's up to you. If you put in the time and make the effort to stay sober and mentally healthy, anything is possible.

Where I live, in Florida, there are many elderly residents. They never seem to be in a hurry. They know how to pace themselves by taking small steps. I'm following their lead. I don't rush or put extra pressure on myself. I'm content to make slow, steady progress. The more I take this approach, the easier and more natural it becomes.

My accomplishments were not made all at once, or even quickly. They're the result of years of slow, steady progress. You have to be patient. The small steps add up. When you make healthy choices over many years, life becomes dramatically better – a step at a time.

Instant success often vanishes as quickly as it appears. Sometimes it's not generally known that an "overnight" success has worked for years to perfect his or her craft. I started writing seriously when I was 12 years old. I first worked with agents and publishers at age 14. It took almost 15 years for a major publisher to purchase the rights to one of my books. Success takes time – sometimes years of slow, steady work. Set big goals for yourself, and work on them with persistence and patience. And don't give up. It will be hard at first but keep going. One day you'll see your investment of time and effort pay off.

Some won't believe in you (or in what you do) for a simple reason: They don't believe in themselves. They worry about what can go wrong and how they'll handle failure.

Believing in yourself means believing in what you do. Would you buy apples from someone who tells you that they don't taste good? I know that I'm a talented therapist and have a lot to share with the world. I accept my ability to achieve, and believe that I deserve the benefits I've earned. I don't need others to tell me this. You need to believe to get started, and you have to continue to believe to keep going. Others will believe when they see your success.

Depression, Bipolar and Heroin

There was a group of crabs in a bucket. When one of the crabs tried to get out, the others stopped him. They were comfortable in the bucket and didn't want anyone to "rock the bucket." They didn't realize that, by escaping, they'd avoid becoming someone's lunch. You may have friends or family members who are like those crabs.

Find a therapist who believes in your potential. When you work with him or her you'll receive real, constructive feedback. When the therapist with whom I worked doubted my goals I quickly found another. Find someone who will mentor, support and help you accomplish your goals. Leave behind the addicts who are holding you back. It won't mean you're a bad person who abandons his/her friends – only that you've realized it's time to save your life. Those addicts know they need to end their addictions too. Your sobriety is like a mirror in front of them, showing them how much they need to change.

Above all, find the version of God in which you believe and develop a relationship with him/her/it. I was born Jewish and consider myself to be a proud Jewish person. This hasn't prevented me from finding strength in other faiths and their leaders. I've learned a lot by listening to Joel Osteen and the Dalai Lama. I consider Joyce Meyer and TD Jakes to be my teachers.

God is the only one who is always there and never fails you. My brother's death was one of the biggest losses I've suffered, but through it all God has been the friend I need. I'm blessed to be able to help you on your journey. As you begin it, I pray that you'll learn, love and grow.

It's time for us to come together and build a world in which we don't lose great people to addiction. A world in which we encourage and support each other. A world in which we deal with our problems in healthy ways. Everyone would find the support they need to find their way back from mental illness and addiction. We'd help each other to live clean lives.

My brother died from his addictions, as have millions of others. He wanted to stop taking drugs, but he didn't know how. I wish I could have saved him and all of your loved ones who died in the same way. But if you and I avoid addiction, we'll live and inspire others.

21: A Final Lesson

Human beings are not meant to live alone. Sadly, many people choose to isolate themselves. They might think that, because of their past or current behavior, they're not worthy of love. They're afraid that others won't understand them or want them around. In the rehab where I worked, many clients told me that they'd get high alone, shooting up in their bedroom, bathroom or garage.

There have been times when I've chosen to be alone. It only made my life harder. Find a few great people to be on your team – family, friends, coaches or anyone who is there to help you. Check out the support groups in your area. *The National Alliance on Mental Illness*, *The Depression and Bipolar Support Alliance*, *Alcoholics Anonymous* and *Narcotics Anonymous* are ready and willing to help you. They have no other interest but to help you deal with the problems you're facing.

Just by being there, I've helped people who struggle with addiction, depression, bipolar disorder, career and relationship problems, loneliness and more. They know that they can reach me whenever they need me – on the phone, or by emailing or texting me. They can also visit my website: **BipolarOnline.com**.

I know how it feels to be afraid to seek help, but I've learned that you need a guide – someone to point you in the right direction and support you along the way. Asking for help is not a sign of weakness. When I get lost while driving, I ask for directions. Sometimes it's best to ask for help from someone who has already been down the road you're traveling. You'll get to where you want to go more quickly and more directly than you would by "winging it" alone.

You don't have to face your problems alone. Begin your recovery with a free session with one of our coaches. No obligation – you decide whether you want to continue working with us for the long term. (Note: Charges will apply if you decide to continue with us after the free session.) We're dedicated to helping you reach your full potential. We care and we listen. We want you to find the confidence and courage to repair your life and live it to the fullest.

We don't offer pipe dreams: all that we do is based on real-life lessons. We provide knowledge that you can use. Most important – you won't be alone anymore. Our coaches will be with you throughout your transition to a better life. Go to **BipolarOnline.com** to learn more about our work.

As a result of the explosion in communications technology, we don't ever have to be alone. We can connect with friends and coaches whenever we like. But connecting will do you good only if you're willing to open up and learn. Some feel they communicate best speaking face to face. Others are comfortable talking on the phone. Me? I love writing. Here's why.

When I left college I found a job as a homeless outreach worker. Each day I drove around Manhattan in a big white van, looking for homeless people. Whenever I saw one or more, I'd park and approach them, ask their names, offer food, and decide whether I could do more to help them. Many were happy just to have someone talk to. Someone who would listen. It wasn't long before I knew most of them by name.

One day I visited a soup kitchen while a book giveaway was in progress. Many of the local homeless people where there, excited by the opportunity to get something to read for free.

Some of those books were 30 or 40 years old, but the people seemed to feel that they were still well worth reading.

When you write, you can connect with readers across great distances, and across the years. I hope that the lessons I share with readers will continue to do good in their lives long after I'm gone. Maybe the example of my brother's death, as I wrote about it in 2014, will help someone in 2114. If it does, his death will have served a higher purpose. I can't bring Adam back, but I can honor him by helping others like him.

Writing these words, and knowing that they'd be read, has helped me to heal. I never felt lower than when I lost Adam, but my inner voice told me to lean on my faith and press on. I can't tell you how happy I am that God chose me to bring this message to you. Out of a dark time, he decided to shine a light of hope for others who face these problems.

The hardest part of losing my brother is knowing that we could have done more together. Much more. I wish he was here to help me with my coaching. I think he would have made a great coach. His final gift was his death, which is a lesson for us all. Don't let what happened to him happen to you. You can defeat your addiction. If you're addicted, seek and accept the help you need. If you aren't, help someone who is.

We are all one people. Each of us is someone's child, and all of us deserve love. You may be ready to live a better life. I promise you that if you begin a journey of healing it will be well worth it. I know why I've experienced so much – good and bad – in my first 35 years of life. All of it, together, has given me the skills I need to positively impact the lives of others. If I continue to help people, God will use me in even greater ways.

You are something wonderful. Believe it. You deserve love, happiness, peace and prosperity. God created you as a gift to the world. Accept that you are special and unique. You don't have to be anyone else. Be yourself. You have gifts that we desperately need.

Thank you for allowing me to share my work with you – I'm honored that you've read my book. Feel free to contact me. Information on how to do so is provided on **BipolarOnline.com**. I'd love to hear whether, and how, what I've written has helped you. Until next time, may God bless you with a wonderful life!

Thank You

I couldn't have written this book without the support of those who encourage and inspire me.

My family is the best part of life. I'm blessed to be married to Jennifer. Her love always keeps me trying to do my best. Our daughter Tyler lights up every room she enters. My son Ryan is bright, curious and loves to smile.

Since I was a boy, my mother has encouraged me to follow my dreams. She's a wonderful therapist who has guided many families towards a better life. My stepfather has accepted the loss of his son, my stepbrother Adam, with grace. Throughout this hard time he's been kind and giving to his grandchildren, and to me. My sister, Chayse, is confident, wise and willing to work for what she believes in. She's remained graceful and poised throughout Adam's death and its aftermath. My grandmother Arlene suffered a severe stroke on the day my brother died, but has worked tirelessly to recover. She's an essential part of our family.

My other dad, Larry, encouraged and supported me through my childhood. My stepmother, Anna, has always been a friend. My stepsister, Natasha, is an excellent student. She's studying to be a teacher. Those who are lucky enough to be her students will receive a great education.

My father-in-law has always been kind and loving to us, helping us through difficult times. My brother-in-law, Scott, is more like a brother to me. He's the same age as Adam – they were close friends. His girlfriend, Martina, works hard to care for her beautiful child and is a loving companion to Scott. I'm happy that they've found each other.

I have a lot of family and friends in the Philadelphia area. My wife and I were married there, and love to go back to visit. My grandpa, Neiman, and his wife, Barbara, live outside the city. They're wonderful grandparents. I love them with all my heart. Their daughters, Jennifer and Danielle, are my amazing aunts. I love laughing and sharing jokes with Jennifer. Danielle is a community leader in Philadelphia who's dedicated to making the city she loves a better place. My daughter loves to spend time with Jennifer's daughters, Lea and Sofia – and so do I. Jennifer's husband Gene is a warm, caring man.

My wife's aunt Sharon and her husband, Avishai, are like parents to us. We love them and their children – Sarah, Asher, Ari, Carly, Sally and David. We're never happier than when we're all together at family gatherings. I also love spending time with Jen's grandmother Bubby, a smart and dynamic woman.

I'll never forget the friends I've made (and what I've learned from them) in Long Island, Manhattan, New Jersey, Los Angeles and Florida. I also want to thank Adam's friends. When he died I met hundreds of them, many whom I'd never met before. They came from all directions to attend his memorial service and celebrate his life. I know he would want me to tell them how much he loved them.

Many books are written by a single author (like this one), but before they're finished many others become involved in doing the work necessary to put them in readers' hands. I feel blessed to have met Tom, my editor, who volunteered to help prepare this book for publication. His kindness helped make it available to you. I also want to thank everyone who has encouraged my writing career. I couldn't have kept going without you. Last of all, I want to thank the patients and clients I've worked with. By sharing the lessons I've learned from you – lessons we learned together – we'll inspire others to seek and find the help they need. Working with you has been a blessing.

Blake LeVine

Words of Wisdom from Blake

If you change, life will change.

Don't give up. Things will get better!

When you help others, you help yourself.

Love is like light. Let it shine.

Learning is the only way to grow.

Your situation is as dark as you make it.

Life is like a game. Keep playing!

Love is everywhere. Do you see it?

Why stay sad when you can be happy?

If today was your last day, what would you do?

Death is not the end, but a new beginning.

Do you see the children, flowers, and sun? If you do, you know life is beautiful.

If you slow down, you'll find peace sooner.

Find what you love to do and do it endlessly.

Whisper kindness into someone's ear. They will come alive.

When will it all change? When you change it.

If you need hope, believe in yourself.

If you quit when things get hard, you won't pass the test.

Don't compare your life to the lives of others. Each has his or her own path.

I've seen joy and pain, and I'll take joy any day.

Let go and choose faith.

God is my best friend, and he knows it.

Loving is winning.

Addiction is a dead end. It leaves you with nowhere to go.

We become addicted to hide. Come out and play.

I wouldn't be alive if I chose to be negative.

Choose hope.

Today is the greatest day of your life.

God believes in you and loves you unconditionally.

Resources

You can't do this alone, and you certainly can't do it if you don't understand what you're up against. Visit the following sites for reliable information about mental illness and addiction.

The National Alliance on Mental Illness	www.nami.org
The Depression and Bipolar Support Alliance	www.dbsalliance.org
Alcoholics Anonymous	www.aa.org
Narcotics Anonymous	www.na.org
International Bipolar Foundation	www.ibpf.org
American Psychiatric Association	www.psych.org
Phoenix House	www.phoenixhouse.org
Partnership for Drug Free Kids	www.drugfree.org
American Society of Addiction Medicine	www.asam.org
Hazelden	www.hazelden.org
National Institute on Drug Abuse	www.drugabuse.gov

National Council on Alcoholism and Drug Dependence	www.ncadd.org
National Institutes of Health	www.nih.gov
The Association for Addiction Professionals	www.naadac.org
The National Association of Social Workers	www.socialworkers.org
American Psychological Association	www.apa.org
American Medical Association	www.ama-assn.org

Books by Blake LeVine

Okay Dad, You Can Take the Picture

Like Mother, Like Son: A Mom's Guide To Raising Healthy Children

Beating Bipolar: How One Therapist Tackled His Illness . . . and How What He Learned Could Help You!

Films by Blake LeVine

Rap Therapy

Online Videos: Youtube.com/willlistenvideos

Blake's Web Sites

www.bipolaronline.com

www.blakespeaking.com

Speaking Events

Blake has spoken about how to overcome addiction and mental illness, and gain a positive outlook, at colleges and corporate locations, at conferences and for professional organizations. To find out how to have Blake speak to your group, visit **www.blakespeaking.com.**

Blake LeVine

About The Author

Blake LeVine is a social worker, life coach and bipolar advocate. As a child, he gained national attention by meeting and interviewing notable people. At age 14 he was invited by President Clinton to visit the White House. As a teenager Blake met Nelson Mandela, Mother Teresa, The Dalai Lama, seven U.S. Presidents, Paul McCartney, Michael Jackson, Princess Diana, Madonna, Audrey Hepburn, Ella Fitzgerald, Steven Spielberg, Bob Dylan, The Rolling Stones, Margaret Thatcher, George Clooney, and over 5,000 other notables.

When he was 15, Blake began to show signs of bipolar disorder. He was diagnosed with bipolar one and spent two years in and out of psychiatric hospitals. He eventually found the right medications and therapy, and began to rebuild his life. He finished high school, graduated from college, and earned a Master's Degree in Social Work.

For over 15 years, Blake has worked as a social worker and life coach. He's helped homeless clients, foster care children, those who suffer from schizophrenia, bipolar disorder, addictions and depression, and cancer survivors. He's appeared on Oprah.com, CNN, Life and Style, BP Magazine and many radio programs, educating audiences about these issues. He also completed a 50-city national media tour on camera with Dr. Drew Pinsky, educating college students about bipolar disorder.

Blake was engaged to his wife on a live broadcast of *The Dr. Phil Show*. They have been happily married for eight years and have two children. He now travels internationally, speaking to a variety of audiences about bipolar disorder. Blake has visited over 30 local chapters of The National Alliance on Mental Illness (NAMI) and The Depression and Bipolar Support Alliance

(DBSA). He wrote *Beating Bipolar*, which was published by Hay House in 2012. Bipolar survivor Demi Lovato publicly praised Blake's book and the work he's done to help others who suffer from this disease.

Blake's goal is to create awareness of bipolar disorder, and to educate people on how to treat it. He has shown that with proper therapy, medications and support groups, those who suffer from it can live healthy lives. He is the founder of **BipolarOnline.com**, where he offers one-on-one coaching, his books, and other resources to those who will benefit from them.

Our Gift to You

If you need additional help we are happy to assist you. **BipolarOnline.com** provides access to coaching and other assistance to those who live with these problems.

We offer one free coaching session to everyone who requests it. Please tell anyone you know who may benefit from a session to contact us for more information. Call us at **(213) 304-9555**, or send email to **blake.levine@aol.com**.

We are also happy to assist you if you would like to write a book – even if you've never written before. We'll help you to get your story down on paper and teach you how to promote it. The world at large benefits when we share our stories and the lessons they've taught us.

If you'd like to contact the author with feedback, questions or for any reason at all, call his office at the number listed above, or send email to the address provided. Thank you for purchasing this book – and reading it! We hope it's been a helpful experience.